THE ARTERIAL ANATOMY OF THE KIDNEY

THE ARTERIAL ANATOMY OF THE KIDNEY

THE BASIS OF SURGICAL TECHNIQUE

BY

F. T. GRAVES, M.S., F.R.C.S.

Urological and Senior Surgeon, Staffordshire General Infirmary Stafford; Lately, Hunterian Professor, Royal College of Surgeons of England

WITH A PROLOGUE BY

SIR ERIC RICHES, M.C., M.S., F.R.C.S.

BALTIMORE: THE WILLIAMS AND WILKINS COMPANY
1971

Distribution by Sole Agents:
United States of America: The Williams & Wilkins Company, Baltimore
Canada: The Macmillan Company of Canada Ltd., Toronto

ISBN 0 7236 0273 5

PRINTED IN GREAT BRITAIN BY HENRY LING LTD., A SUBSIDIARY OF JOHN WRIGHT & SONS LTD., AT THE DORSET PRESS, DORCHESTER

TO

MARY, DOROTHY, AND JOHN

CONTENTS

THE PROLOGUE

SIX centuries ago Geoffrey Chaucer wrote the Prologue to the *Canterbury Tales* to explain the reasons for the pilgrimage and the circumstances attending its inauguration. He introduced the characters but left them to tell their own stories in turn. The motive for this book is described in the first chapter; it sprang from the notion that removal of the whole kidney should not be necessary if only a fraction of it is diseased. The story of the investigation of the problem is given in the subsequent chapters; unlike the disconnected individual tales of Chaucer's pilgrims they are arranged in orderly and logical sequence to emphasize their dependence on one another. The solution of the problem was seen at once to be in an exact knowledge of anatomy, in particular the detailed anatomy of the renal arterial system. William Hunter in his plea to the government in 1763 said 'Anatomy is the only solid foundation of medicine. It is to the physician and surgeon what geometry is to the astronomer'. John Hunter, who had learned his anatomy by dissecting for his brother William, had noted in 1794 that there was no anastomosis of the arteries supplying the different areas of the kidney. This observation was omitted from textbooks of anatomy even in the present century. Its confirmation was the second object of the research here described, the first being to determine whether there was a constancy of pattern of the arteries to the kidney. The linkage of these two factors has given information of great surgical significance.

The investigation has been carried out in true Hunterian manner, by experiment and observation. Facts are important, not unconfirmed opinions.

Although some of the present information has already been published in separate articles, it has now been revised and amplified in greater detail so that it forms a unified and convenient work of reference for urological and general surgeons and their pupils, as well as for anatomists. Its ultimate aim is to clarify and improve renal surgery and to this end a completely new chapter on surgical technique has been added. Teachers of anatomy will find that stress has been laid on those anatomical points which have a direct bearing on surgery; this is of particular importance now that the time for dissection in the medical student's curriculum has been drastically curtailed.

The chief method of investigation used was to inject the renal arteries of fresh autopsy kidneys with a resin which could be coloured and which would harden in a predetermined time according to its exact composition and temperature. The pelvi-calicine system was injected with resin of a different colour. The organic material of the kidney was then removed by immersion in strong hydrochloric acid. The resultant specimen was a cast showing the renal arteries and their relation to the pelvis and calices. Many such casts were studied. Full details of the preparation of the resin and the techniques of injection and corrosion are given so that others with the requisite patience and industry can repeat the experiments if they so desire.

Injections of anatomical specimens had been done by the Hunters, and William had studied the methods of Frank Nichols in London in 1741 and of Albinus in Leyden in 1748; the difference now lies in the more scientific choice of the materials and the complete destruction of the surrounding tissues which has made accurate study possible. The results of Graves' study show that the kidney is divisible into five segments, each with its own artery arising from either the anterior or the posterior division of the main renal artery. There are some variations in the site of origin of the segmental arteries which can be classified into three groups; these are of surgical importance. There are also variations in the origin of the apical segment artery which fall into four types; these are of less importance to the surgeon but he must remember that the apical segment artery, like that to the lower segment, supplies both the anterior and posterior surfaces of the corresponding kidney segment. Study of casts made by selective segment injection shows conclusively that there is no collateral circulation between one segmental artery and another; they are end arteries. The conclusions have been substantiated by other experiments, including renal arteriography.

When similar experiments were repeated in the renal veins it was found that there was no segmental arrangement but a free anastomosis of all the venous channels of the kidney. The vexed problem of 'aberrant' and 'accessory' renal arteries is convincingly explained; they are normal segmental vessels but with an abnormal point of origin from the aorta or an abnormal site of entry into the kidney, at the pole instead of the hilum.

In the kidney which is congenitally abnormal, whether in site, fusion, duplicity, or pelvis, the apparent variations in its arterial supply still fall into an ordered pattern. The explanation of multiple renal arteries demands a knowledge of the development of the mesonephric arteries—some persist and some degenerate. There is still no collateral circulation between them in the kidney.

Some kidneys containing cysts, tumours, or stones have also been studied. The 'pooling' in arteriograms of renal tumours is considered to be due to delayed emptying of the intrarenal veins due to their partial obstruction by growth. In calculous disease there is little change in the distribution or calibre of the arteries, but some loss of pattern of the finer cortical vessels. There are some interesting observations on the mode of formation of renal calculi.

For the surgeon all the detailed anatomical knowledge of the arteries reaches its acme in the operation of partial nephrectomy, for which there are many indications; the technique advised is described in detail. It must be remembered that only the apical or the lower segment can be completely deprived of its arterial supply by division of its segmental artery. In resection of the lower pole it is important to see whether the middle and lower segment arteries arise from a common stem (Group II) and, if so, to ligate the lower segment artery distal to the origin of that to the middle segment. The origin of the ovarian or testicular artery must also be seen as it may arise from the artery to the lower segment, especially if that artery springs directly from the aorta. In resection of the upper pole, division of the upper segment artery will not render the posterior surface bloodless, as it is supplied by the posterior segment artery. This passes behind the neck of the upper calix and is at risk in upper pole resection; its division will render a large area of the posterior surface of the kidney avascular. It is here that the method of serial section described has its greatest value, but adequate exposure and display of the vessels is the greatest safeguard.

The removal of a large staghorn calculus can be facilitated by resection of the upper or lower poles, or of both; osteotomy of the neck of the horn of the stone may be necessary. The operation can be aided by local renal hypothermia of which a full description is given; the kidney is cooled in a plastic bag by a sterilized solution of cold antifreeze (30 per cent glycerine in water). The results of this procedure in 52 patients, including some with a solitary kidney, are summarized; there were no deaths and no postoperative urological complications.

This book is written in a philosophical style and is easy to read. The numerous illustrations add to the vitality of the text and enhance its value to the student. The colour photographs of casts, the work of John Graves, are of great beauty and clarity.

It was said of Chaucer's Clerk that 'Gladly wolde he lerne, and gladly teche'. This could well apply to the author.

ERIC RICHES

THE ARTERIAL ANATOMY OF THE KIDNEY

CHAPTER ONE

INTRODUCTION

It was a hot summer's afternoon in 1952. A bluebottle buzzed intermittently outside the theatre window, and beyond, the patchwork quilt of London's roof-land simmered in a smoky haze towards St. Paul's and the horizon.

Behind me the surgical team had completed their preliminary manœuvres and the operation had started. I turned to watch. The problem was not uncommon; the patient had a stone of a fair size, embedded in the lower calix of the kidney. Both kidneys were otherwise normal and had good function. As the operation progressed the kidney was exposed and, in order to locate the stone, the surgeon took a blunt needle and passed it gently through the solid substance of the kidney until he felt the grating of the stone upon the metal. Having found it, he incised the cortex and cut down upon the stone, which he then removed.

A simple operation. A standard procedure.

One day, a fortnight later, I heard one of my colleagues say that in the post-operative period the patient had lost so much blood by persistent bleeding into the urine that a second operation had become necessary, at which the kidney was removed.

A month later the same procedure was carried out by a different surgeon on another patient who, by some ill fate, also suffered extreme blood-loss in the postoperative period, so that the affected kidney had to be removed at a second operation in order to save his life.

This strange coincidence of misfortune in which two patients had had to lose what was, in fact, a perfectly normal kidney, apart from the presence of a stone, provoked much thought in my mind. It would not perhaps have been so bad if the whole kidney had been diseased, but when only a fraction of it was affected, then the sacrifice of the remainder seemed a heavy price to pay. The surgeon, however, had had little option for the patient was bleeding, his life was in the balance, and the kidney on the other side would carry the load.

Nevertheless it seemed to me an extraordinary thing that in the piping days of peace of 1952, we knew so little about where the blood-vessels lay within the substance of the kidney—so little indeed that any incision made might, by chance, produce a torrential haemorrhage, or at best a chronic blood-loss.

At this time I was a Registrar working on a Thoracic Unit. Much of my 'spare time' was spent in the study of the bronchial tree and vessels, together with the segmental anatomy of the lung, which had recently been described by Sir Russell Brock.

One day the thought struck me. Had anyone ever studied or described the arterial pattern within the substance of the kidney? Could there be any segmental arrangement in the same way that had been found in the lung? Other questions followed quickly on. I embarked on a search of the literature of the present half-century but this produced no evidence that the anatomy of the intrarenal vessels had been studied to any extent. In 1901 Max Brodel had advocated an incision on the posterior side of the lateral border of the kidney, as this site was thought to be relatively avascular. In practice, however, most surgeons had found that this proved to be by no means a bloodless area.

Enquiry into the less numerous but more descriptive journals and textbooks of the era from 1900 back to 1850 brought similar negative results. Most of the textbooks referred to 'the arcuate arteries of the kidney', and implied that there was a series of arterial arcades which produced a free anastomosis throughout the kidney. There was, however, little or no description of how such evidence was obtained, and indeed I obtained the impression that there was a tendency for diagrams to be copied from one generation to another.

It was not until I chanced upon the writings of John Hunter, one dull autumn afternoon, that I found a glimmering of truth, for in 1794 he wrote 'The veins in the spleen and kidneys anastomose in very large trunks, while the arteries do not at all'.

A man of purpose was John Hunter. 'Boldness and independence in the pursuit of truth was one of the striking characteristics of Hunter's mind. He attached no value to opinions but only to facts. Instead, therefore, of referring to the discoveries detailed in books, he appealed directly to Nature herself until, by the evidence of his own senses, he had ascertained the truth.'

Like John Hunter it seemed that I, too, must appeal unto Nature, for the need for information was of obvious importance. The facts could only be found by experiment.

CHAPTER TWO

THE EXPERIMENTS

BASIC PRINCIPLES

IN planning the investigation it was essential to follow three basic principles: to remain impartial from previous knowledge and to accept only those facts which could be proved by experiment; secondly, to decide at the outset of the investigation, or at each stage, specific questions for which the research must provide an answer; and lastly to develop techniques which, as far as possible, would produce no pitfalls to distort the assessment of the results of the work.

The first stage of the research was therefore planned and carried out in order to answer the following questions:—

1. Is there a constant pattern of the branches of the renal artery within the substance of the kidney?
2. If the pattern is constant, is there a collateral circulation between these branches?
3. Could knowledge of the two previous points be applied to surgery, and in particular to a segmental resection of the kidney?

METHODS OF INVESTIGATION

As the kidney has an insular circulation the obvious method of investigation was to inject the renal artery with some substance which would take up the shape and pattern of the arterial vessels so that these would remain for examination after the organic material had been removed. Previous investigators had used various substances for injection, including red lead and gelatine, but these had had many disadvantages, one of which had been that often the medium had to be injected under considerable pressure in order to ensure that it reached the smaller vessels. This, I felt, was of particular disadvantage since unusual pressure might force the medium into abnormal tissues or planes and give the false impression of the existence of channels which in fact did not exist in the natural state.

Post-mortem specimens of the human kidney were used throughout my investigations. As it was found that the main stem of the renal artery divides into its branches at any point between the hilum and the aorta, it was essential to take a block of tissue, including the kidney and its surrounding fat, together with the adjacent part of the aorta. Only by so doing could it be certain that all vessels entering the kidney would be included in the cast. One further point: it was also important to avoid dissection of vessels in the neighbourhood of the renal artery or hilum lest the very vessels which were being investigated were damaged at the outset of the experiment.

In view of the previous considerations I decided to carry out the first stage of the investigation by injecting the renal artery of a post-mortem kidney with a liquid plastic material, and subsequently to remove the organic material of the kidney by a process of corrosion in an acid bath.

Injection of Post-mortem Specimens with Plastic

A Marco Resin was injected.* This is an unsaturated polyester which is a distinct grouping of resinous compounds formed by the reaction between a polyhydric alcohol and a polybasic acid, one of which contains the unsaturated group —CH= CH—. Such an ester remains unsaturated and because of the shape and size of the molecules, the unsaturated groupings do not come into contact with resultant chemical combination.

This non-reactivity of the double bond can be changed by the addition of a substance called a 'modifying monomer' which, in the presence of a suitable catalyst, will convert the polyester resin from its consistency of a resinous syrup to a hard and slightly elastic solid. Unsaturated polyester resins can be cast quite easily at room temperature and be made to set in times varying between a few minutes and several hours.

A standard polyester resin was used at first but this was not found to be very satisfactory. After some experimentation a resin of a different formula was used at the suggestion of the manufacturers (Marco Resin, S.B. 61c) and this was found to be an excellent medium for the investigation. In making the choice of a resin a number of criteria have to be considered. The resin in its liquid state must not be too viscous, otherwise its capacity to permeate the smaller capillaries is impaired. The capacity of the resin to set must not be inhibited by the presence of water, blood, or any other impurities in the specimen. Lastly the resistance of the resin, once it had set, to the action of hydrochloric acid must be high, otherwise the cast would tend to be destroyed when the organic material was removed by the action of the acid in the corrosive bath.

After experimentation, using benzoyl peroxide as the catalyst, it was found that the liquid resin would set within 10–20 minutes after injection into the blood-vessels if the following proportions were used:—

Resin S.B. 61c	12·5 g.
Monomer 'C'	2·0 g.
Benzoyl peroxide	0·35 g.

The rate of setting, using these proportions, depended slightly upon the surrounding temperature, a higher temperature causing the resin to set more quickly. Over a narrow range setting could be hastened by increasing the amount of the catalyst. Excess catalyst, however, or alternatively too little catalyst, resulted in complete failure of the resin to solidify.

Resin S.B. 61c was used in the making of almost all the casts in this work. The resin has, however, now been superseded by Scott Bader Resin 'Crystic 700' which is a water-clear unsaturated polyester resin for which the manufacturers recommend the following formula for casting:—

Crystic 700	100 parts by weight
Monomer 'C'	20 parts by weight
Catalyst paste H	4 parts by weight
Pigment or dye	4 parts by weight
Accelerator E	0·5–2 parts by weight

*Polyester resin was supplied by Scott Bader & Co. Ltd., Wollaston, Wellingborough, Northamptonshire.

A word of caution is essential. It is vital to mix the ingredients in the order recommended by the manufacturers, and of particular importance that the catalyst and accelerator should not be mixed directly with each other, since they can react with explosive violence. The liquid Crystic 700 is inflammable and must be kept away from naked flames.

Preparation of the Resin for Injection

Using the Resin S.B. 61c, the catalyst, benzoyl peroxide, was ground to a fine powder in a beaker, with some caution; to a fine powder since the presence of a large granule of catalyst remaining undissolved in the final mixture of resin occasionally caused the cast to break at the site of the granule; with caution as benzoyl peroxide is a powerful oxidizing agent, and is potentially explosive. In practice, however, and by using small quantities, no mishaps occurred.

To the powdered catalyst was added a small quantity of colouring matter and to this, in turn, the Monomer 'C'. Finally the whole was added to the resin and mixed, both quickly and thoroughly. The mixing was done by a glass rod in a small glass beaker. Experience taught one that after about 40 seconds there was a subtle change in the consistency of the mixture which indicated that chemical combination was taking place and the resin was ready for use.

Injection Technique

Only fresh specimens of kidneys from the operation theatre or the post-mortem room were used. The use of specimens which had been preserved in formaldehyde or other preservative was not satisfactory. If specimens became available at a time when it was inconvenient to carry out the injection with the resin, the kidneys were stored in a polythene bag in the 'deep freeze' for an almost indefinite period until such time as they could be investigated.

First a cannula was tied into the renal artery through the lumen of the aorta, and at the same time any other vessels arising from the aorta which might possibly enter the renal substance were also cannulated. Secondly the arterial or venous system, whichever was under investigation, was irrigated with warm water by use of a 10- or 20-ml. syringe, in order to dispel such blood as remained in the specimen. If the kidney specimens had been stored in the 'deep freeze,' they were allowed to reach room temperature before the injection was carried out.

The prepared resin was then poured into a clinical syringe and injected into the renal artery and its associated vessels, which were immediately ligated after completing the injection and withdrawing the cannula. By the same technique a similar quantity of a resin of a different colour was injected into the pelvi-calicine system.

There are a few practical points of importance. In general 5–10 ml. of resin were injected, depending on the size of the kidney. Too little resin produced a cast whose vessels were inadequately filled; too much produced a heavy deposit of resin in the cortex, or else gave rise to bursting of the smaller vessels. As the resin, once mixed with the monomer and catalyst, sets quite quickly, one has to be fairly quick with the injection, otherwise the resin may set in the syringe or before injection is complete. For this reason it is wise to attempt only the injection of one specimen at a time until, as says Hippocrates 'one is proficient in the art'.

I found in practice that it was quite unnecessary to use complicated systems with manometers and gauges to control the pressure of injection. A gentle but steady pressure on the syringe produced an even injection of whatever system was being investigated, without fuss and bother. Excess pressure could, however, especially in kidneys affected by arteriosclerosis, sometimes produce extravasation of the resin into abnormal planes, or produce small dissection leaks where there were atheromatous plaques in the main vessels.

Lastly it must be remembered that the resin, during the process of setting to the solid state, undergoes chemical combination and gives out a quantity of heat.

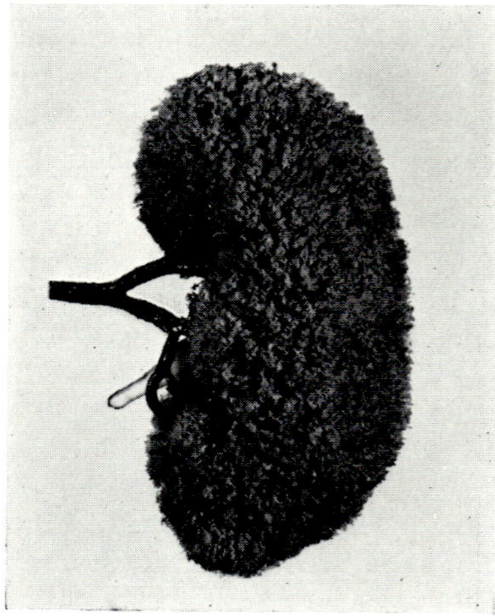

FIG. 1.—A cast of the left kidney seen from the front. The resin has filled all the arterial vessels, including the capillaries of the glomeruli.

With simple injections this is of little consequence, for the heat is easily dispelled through the specimen. If, however, a large quantity of resin is collected in a cavity (as for instance in a cyst) the heat produced can be quite considerable, and as a result the whole cast may split. To avoid such exothermic cracking it is best to fill the cavity in layers, allowing each layer to set, before adding the next.

When the resin had set, the specimen was placed in a bath of concentrated hydrochloric acid, so that the organic substance of the kidney would gradually be removed by corrosion, leaving a cast of the arterial system. Final clearing of the cast was done by washing in warm water and subsequent rinsing of the cast for a brief period in a mixture of equal parts of acetone and ether to remove fatty substances. (The resin is to some extent soluble in acetone if left for a long period of some hours.)

Examination of the Casts

The arterial systems of all the specimens were injected to their full capacity, with the result that each specimen, on being taken from the acid bath, had an appearance not unlike that of a sponge (*Fig.* 1).

In one or two specimens the resin had permeated the fine vessels sufficiently for casts of the glomerular tufts to be seen with the aid of a hand lens. As this fine 'fluff' produced by the casts of the glomeruli obscured the anatomical detail of the larger vessels and their branches, it was removed by hand picking with a fine wire.

CHAPTER THREE

ANATOMY AND NOMENCLATURE

CASTS were made of more than forty specimens of normal human kidneys. On the basis of the arterial distribution it was discovered from the examination of the casts that the kidney was divisible into five segments (*Fig.* 2).

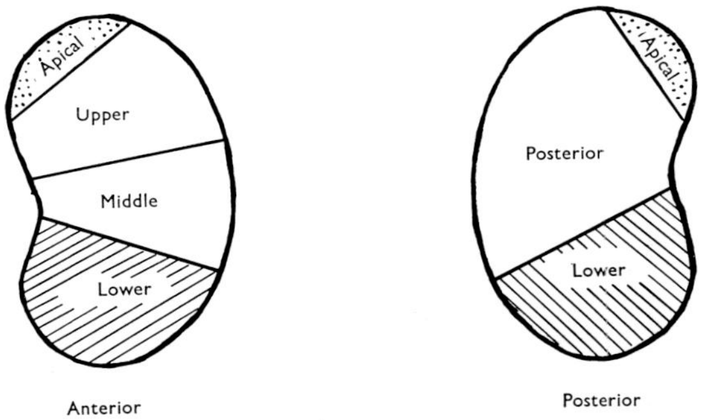

FIG. 2.—A diagram of the left kidney showing the segments which are based on the arterial distribution. Only the apical and lower segments occupy areas on both the anterior and posterior planes of the kidney.

From above downwards these are:—

The apical segment is a cap of tissue which occupies the medial side of the upper pole of the kidney—mainly on its anterior surface.

The upper (*anterior*) *segment* lies in the anterior plane of the kidney. It covers an area which includes the upper pole and part of the central area of the kidney.

The middle (*anterior*) *segment* lies in the anterior plane of the kidney. It covers an area in the lower central part, between the upper and lower segments.

The lower segment forms the lower pole of the kidney. Unlike the middle and upper segments, it lies in both the anterior and posterior planes of the kidney.

The posterior segment lies entirely in the posterior plane of the kidney and occupies an area between the posterior part of the apical segment above, and the posterior portion of the lower segment below.

ANATOMY OF THE RENAL ARTERIES WITHIN THE KIDNEY

Each segment is supplied by its own artery (*Figs.* 3–5). The main stem of the renal artery divides at a variable point between the aorta and the hilum of the kidney into an anterior and posterior division.

The *anterior division* gives rise to the upper, middle, and lower segment arteries, and the apical segment artery usually arises from it.

The *posterior division* continues and supplies only the posterior segment, but it may give origin to the artery to the apical segment.

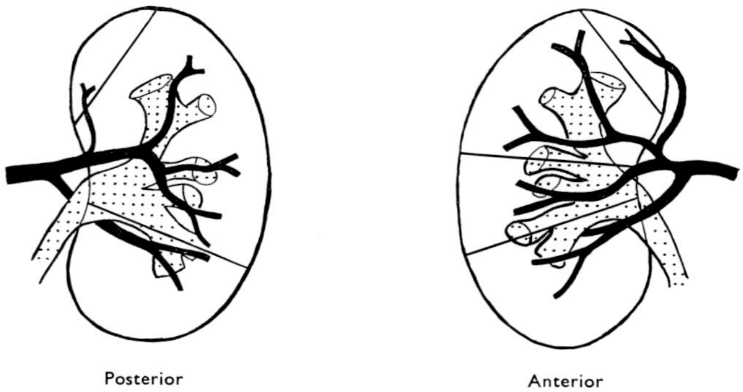

FIG. 3.—A diagram of the right kidney showing the arrangement of the arteries and the segments they supply. The artery to the apical segment is that of Type I. The arrangement of the remaining anterior segment arteries is that of Group I. Compare with *Figs.* 4 and 7.

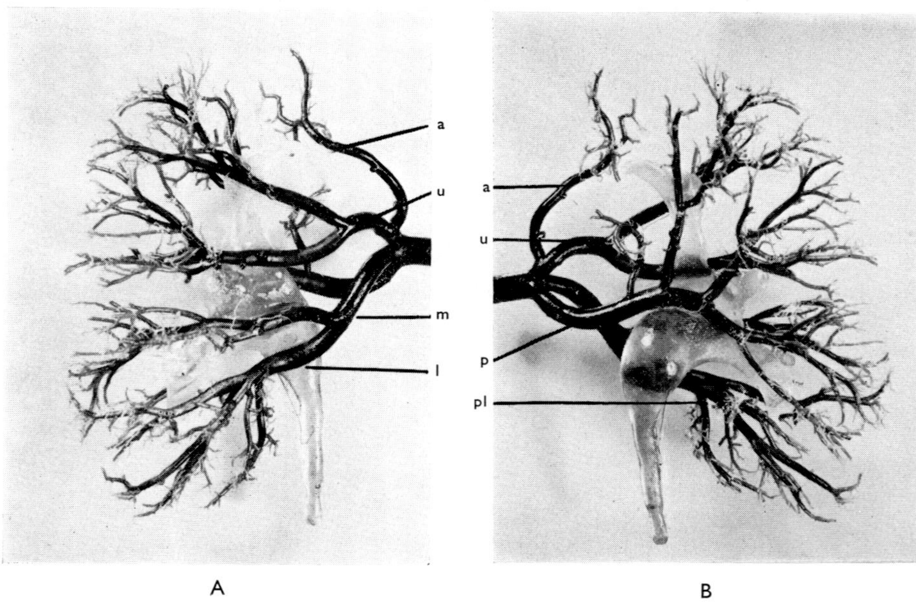

FIG. 4.—A cast of the right kidney. A is labelled to indicate the apical (a), upper (u), middle (m), and lower (l) segment arteries. The apical segment artery arises from the artery to the upper segment; the middle segment artery arises from the side of the lower segment artery, as in Group II. B shows the posterior view of the same cast. Note the course of the posterior segment artery (p) as it courses close to the superior pelvi-calicine junction; note also the posterior branch of the lower segment artery (pl), which supplies the posterior part of the lower pole. See also *Fig.* 5.

THE SEGMENTAL ARTERIES

The Apical Segment Artery

The apical segment is supplied by an artery which most frequently arises from the anterior division. It is, however, a vessel whose origin is the most varied of all the

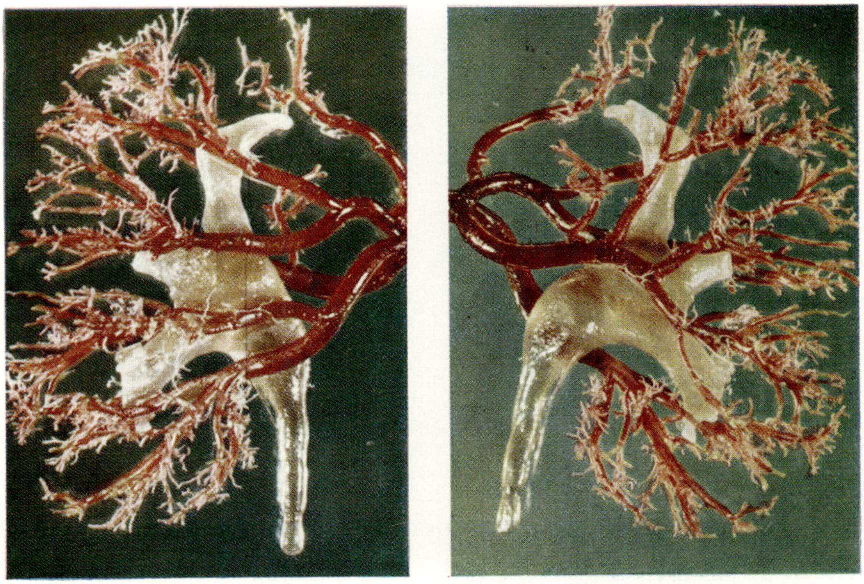

FIG. 5.—A photograph of the same cast of the right kidney seen in *Fig.* 4. The colour indicates more clearly the distribution of the arterial pattern. A, The cast seen from the front; B, The cast seen from behind.

segmental arteries. In order of frequency it arises from the short trunk of the anterior division or the upper segment artery; from the junction of the anterior

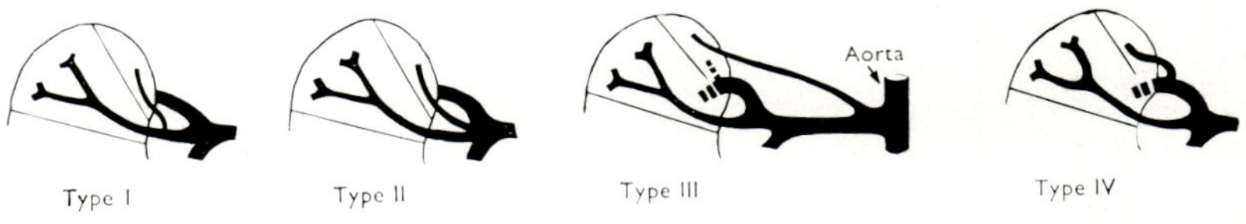

FIG. 6.—A diagram of the variations of origin of the artery to the apical segment in a right kidney. Type I, It arises from the upper segment artery. Type II, It arises from the junction of the anterior and posterior divisions with the main-stem artery. Type III, It arises near the aorta and makes an extrahilar entry to its segment. There is a small accessory artery to the segment arising from the posterior division. Type IV, It arises from the posterior division.

and posterior divisions with the main stem; from the main stem or the aorta; from the posterior division (*Fig.* 6).

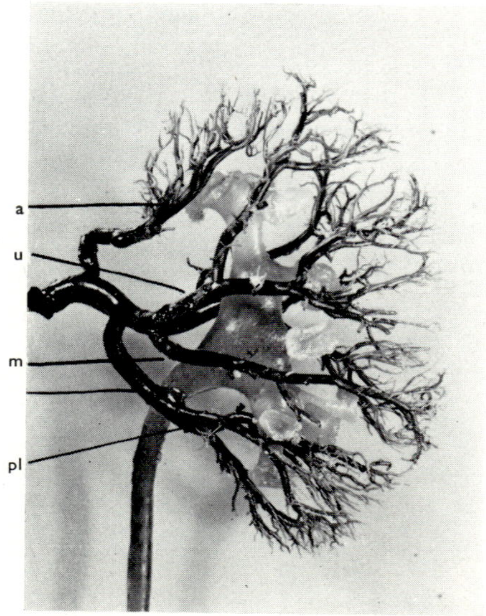

FIG. 7.—A cast of the left kidney seen from the front. The arrows indicate the apical (a), upper (u), middle (m), and lower (l) segment arteries. Note the posterior branch of the lower segment artery (pl) as it passes behind the inferior calix. The apical segment arises from the anterior division. The origins of the remaining anterior segment arteries are as in Group I. See also *Fig.* 8.

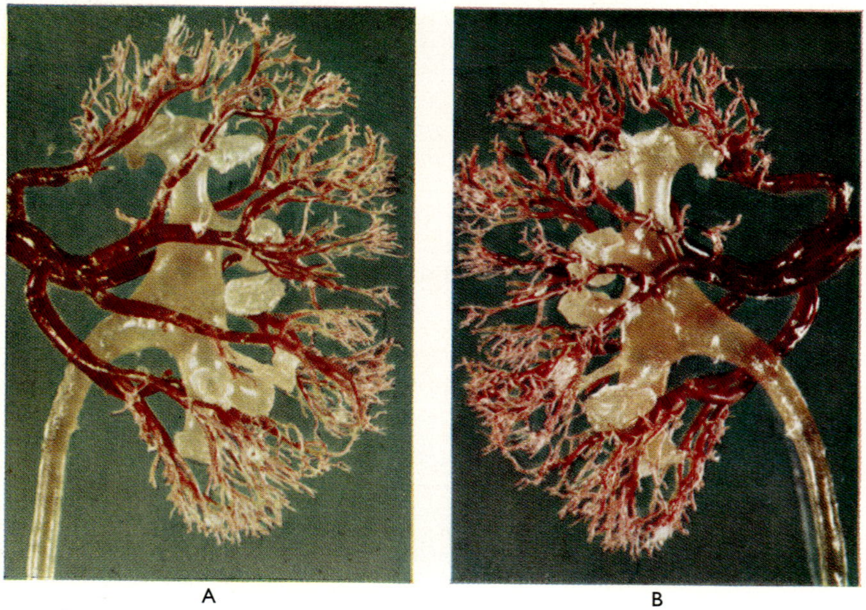

FIG. 8.—The same cast of the left kidney shown in *Fig.* 7, but photographed in colour to show more clearly the detail of the arterial pattern. A, The cast seen from the front; B, The cast seen from behind. B shows the posterior branch of the lower segment artery, very clearly, as it passes behind the inferior calix to supply the posterior aspect of the lower pole.

TYPE I

In 43·3 per cent of cases the artery arises from the trunk of the anterior division or the artery to the upper segment (*Figs.* 7, 8). If it arises from the anterior division its point of origin is easily seen in the hilum well away from the solid substance of the kidney. If it arises as a branch of the upper segment artery, its point of origin may be seen in the hilum, under the lip of the hilum, or more rarely within the parenchyma.

TYPE II

In 23·3 per cent of cases the artery arises from the junction of the anterior and posterior divisions with the main stem. This point of origin is either in the hilum or nearer the aorta. The vessel enters its segment usually from the anterior aspect of the hilum (*see Fig.* 19, p. 22).

TYPE III

In 23·3 per cent of cases the artery arises from the main stem or the aorta itself. The artery runs with its fellows to the hilum, or it may make an extrahilar entry

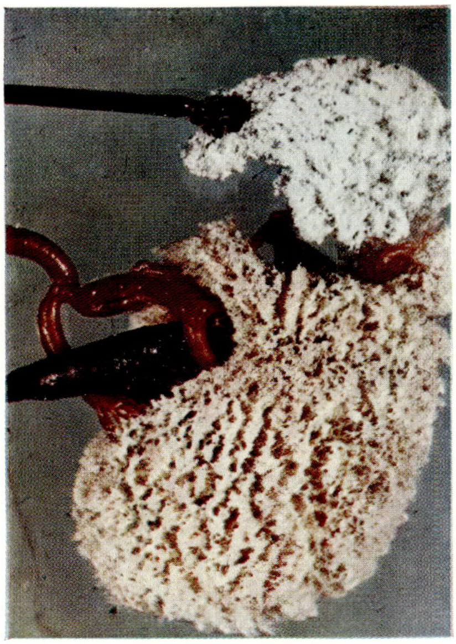

FIG. 9.—The posterior view of a cast of the right kidney. The artery to the apical segment arises directly from the aorta and makes an extrahilar entry to its segment. It has been injected with blue resin. The specimen has been mounted with some displacement in order to show the outline of the segment. The remainder of the kidney has been injected with red resin. Note the clearly defined difference in colour between the areas.

i1 to the side of its segment and in this respect may have the appearance of an 'aberrant' or 'accessory' artery. In this series of specimens about one-third of this type had an extrahilar entry, most of the vessels having arisen directly from the aorta (*Figs.* 9, 10).

Type IV

In 10 per cent of cases the artery arises from the posterior division and enters the segment from the posterior aspect of the hilum (*Fig.* 11).

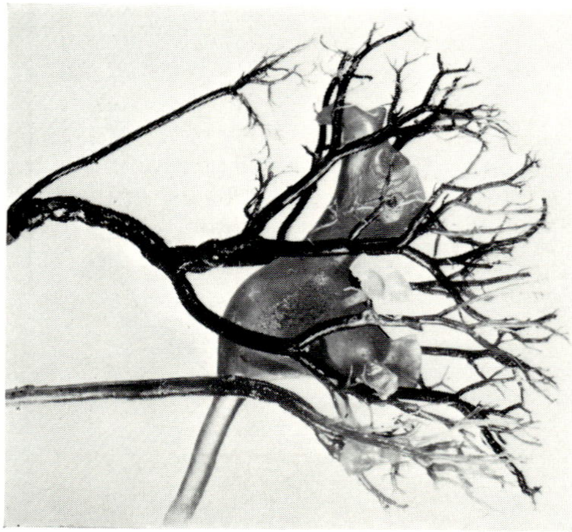

Fig. 10.—A cast of the left kidney seen from the front. The apical segment artery arises from the point of origin of the main stem from the aorta, and makes an extrahilar entry to its segment. There is a small accessory apical segment artery, which arises from the artery to the upper segment. The artery to the lower segment arises directly from the aorta and has been injected with a resin of lighter colour, the arrangement of the anterior segment arteries being as in Group I.

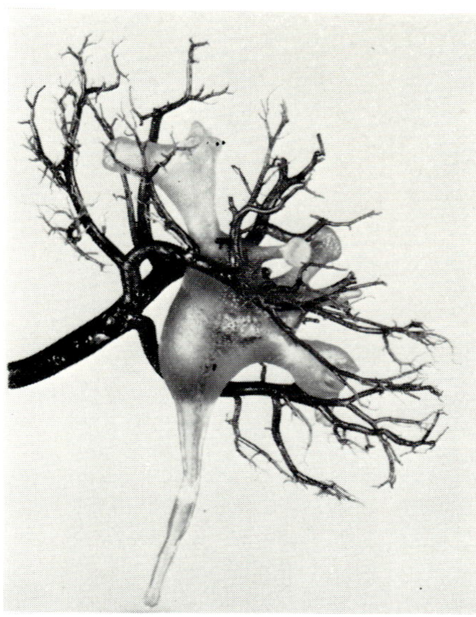

Fig. 11.—The posterior view of a cast of the right kidney. The artery to the apical segment is large and arises from the posterior division as in Type IV.

Accessory Apical Segment Artery

In one-third of the specimens there is a small accessory artery to the apical segment which frequently originates from the posterior division and enters the segment from that aspect. Accessory vessels are present mainly in two types of cases:—

a. In those where the main apical artery enters the segment 'high up', that is an extrahilar entry, and thereby leaves a small area between the point of entry and the base of the segment which is supplied by the accessory vessel.

b. In those cases where both the artery to the upper segment and the artery to the apical segment lie nearer the lateral border of the kidney, a small area is left on the posteromedial side which is supplied by the accessory vessel (*see Figs.* 10, 13).

The Upper Segment Artery

This arises from the anterior division and enters the segment at its base. Its point of origin is usually in the hilum, or under the hilar lip, and can be seen easily. Soon after its entry into the segment, it divides usually into two branches: an apical branch which runs upwards and lies in front of the upper calix and a lateral branch which runs laterally to supply the lateral border of the kidney. The presence and size of these two branches depends largely upon the size and shape of the upper calix. If the pelvi-caliceal system is long and narrow, both branches are well formed (*see Figs.* 7, 8A), but where there are only small middle calices or the artery to the middle segment is big, then the lateral branch is usually small.

The Middle Segment Artery

This arises from the anterior division. If the middle calices are present, it supplies the kidney substance on their anterior aspect, its terminal branches interdigitating with those from the posterior division. If the upper and lower major calices are large, and there are no middle calices, then the middle segment and its artery are correspondingly small, the latter supplying the 'gap' between the two major calices.

The Lower Segment Artery

This artery arises from the anterior division. It passes usually in front of the pelvis or ureter and soon after its entry into the segment it divides into an anterior and posterior branch. The presence and course of these two branches is so constant that the lower pole of a cast or an arteriogram can always be recognized by it (*see Figs.* 4B, 7, 8B).

The anterior branch divides and supplies the anterior aspect of the lower calix and the tip of the lower pole. The posterior branch passes under the neck of the lower calix and supplies the posterior and lower aspect of the lower pole.

The Posterior Segment Artery

This is the continuation of the posterior division. It enters the posterior aspect of the hilum running from front to back across the upper border of the pelvis of the kidney. It then passes behind and in close association with the junction of the upper calix and the pelvis; this relationship is a constant landmark (*see Figs.* 4B, 8B, 13B). The artery runs under the lip of the hilum and forms a curve from whose lateral border branches radiate outwards and enter the segment. (This probably corresponds to that described by Albarran (1909) as 'l'artère retro-pyelique'.) The branches form three groups:—

a. An upper group of one or two in number which supply the posterior part of the upper calix. If there is one vessel only it is often large.

b. A middle group which is usually small and interdigitates with those of the middle segment from the anterior division.

c. A terminal group, branches of which supply the upper part of the lower calix on its posterior surface, the area being larger when the posterior branch of the lower segment artery is small.

VARIATIONS IN THE ARTERIAL PATTERN

In this series of casts the presence of individual segmental arteries has been constant. The only variation has been one of size (usually related to the variation in the size of the segment concerned), and of the exact point of origin of the artery from the main stem.

Variations in the Origins of the Segmental Arteries

The main stem artery divides into an anterior and posterior division at any point between the aorta and the hilum. The posterior division continues as the artery to the posterior segment and has no further variation in its course or origin.

The variations in the origin of the artery to the apical segment have been described. It is with the remaining segmental arteries, the upper, middle, and lower

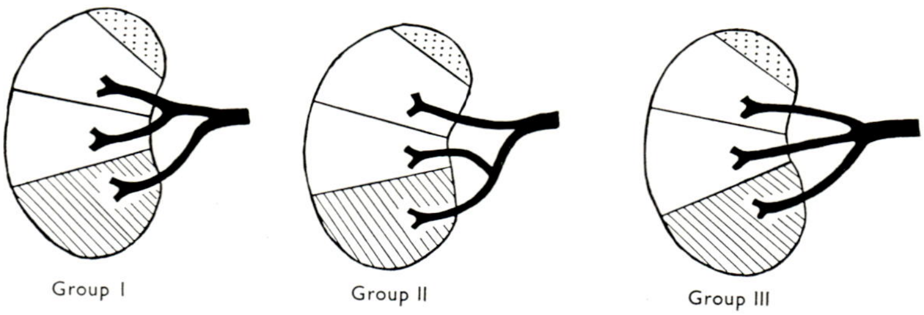

Fig. 12.—A diagram of the right kidney showing the variation in origin of the upper, middle, and lower segment arteries from the anterior division.

arteries of the anterior division, that variations occur. These variations fall into three groups (*Fig.* 12).

Group I

The lower artery arises first; the upper and middle arteries have a common origin. The artery to the lower segment may originate at any point between the hilum and the aorta, or it may arise separately from the aorta a little below the origin of the main stem. This group is the most common. It occurs in 53·3 per cent of cases. (*See Figs.* 7, 8A).

Group II

The lower artery arises with, or more usually a little proximal to the upper artery. The middle artery arises from the side of the lower artery. This is the next most common group, occurring in 30 per cent of cases (*see Figs.* 4A, 5A).

Group III

The lower, middle, and upper segmental arteries have their origin at a common point. This group occurs in 16·6 per cent of cases (*Fig.* 13A).

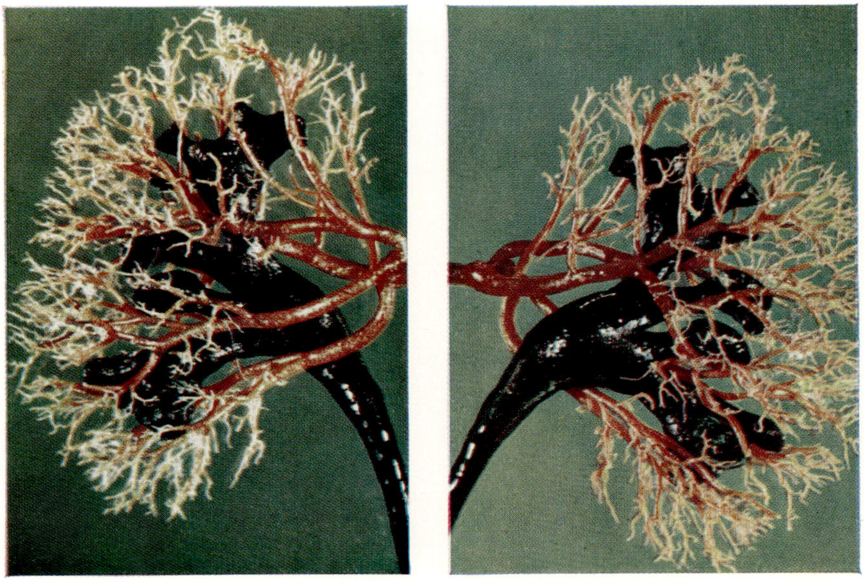

A B

FIG. 13.—Photographs of a cast of the right kidney. A, The cast seen from the front; B, The posterior view. The apical and lateral branches of the upper segment artery are well developed. The origins of the anterior segment arteries are as in Group III. The apical segment artery arises from the posterior division.

INVESTIGATION OF CIRCULATION BETWEEN ARTERIAL SEGMENTS

The investigations described in the previous paragraphs have shown that the arterial pattern within the substance of the kidney is not only reasonably constant, but is found to consist of well-marked and easily discernible segments. In some of the earlier editions of textbooks of anatomy and histology there is mention of 'arciform' and also of 'arcuate arteries' which tends to suggest that there may be a free anastomosis between the smaller arteries of the kidney. The question as to whether there is or is not a collateral arterial circulation between different segments of the kidney is of considerable importance, partly from the viewpoint of surgery, and partly from the aspect of pathology, since a free anastomosis between segments would lessen the possibility of infarction occurring, in the event of a blockage of a segmental artery, either by surgical ligation or by pathological accident.

An investigation was therefore carried out, by four different methods, to determine whether there was any collateral circulation between the arterial segments. The first of these, however, arose by 'accident' more than design and, in fact, it was this casual observation which stimulated more detailed enquiry.

FIRST EXPERIMENT

During the previous investigations it was noticed that one of the post-mortem specimens of the kidney had been inadvertently damaged in the process of its removal from the cadaver, with the result that the lower segment artery had been severed from the main renal vessel. Although it was therefore of no use for the investigation being carried out at the time, it was nevertheless injected with resin as a matter of interest. I injected the main renal artery with a red resin, and as it was getting late at night, rather than mix further resin I injected the lower segment

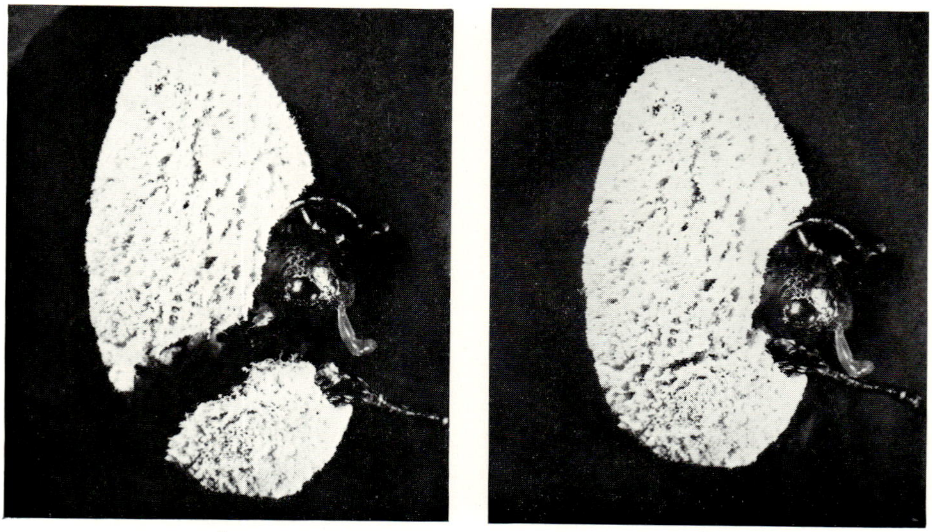

A B

FIG. 14.—A, The cast of the lower segment which has become separated from the rest of the cast of the kidney whilst in the acid bath. B, The separated segment, after being replaced in the main cast.

artery with a small quantity of resin of the same colour which had been left unused. I then withdrew the cannulae, after ligating the vessels in the usual way, and placed the kidney in the corrosive acid bath.

Some days later, when the cast was taken from the acid bath, I noticed that the lower segment was missing. A search in the acid, however, produced the complete cast of the lower segment, which had fallen apart from the main cast when the supporting organic tissue of the kidney had been removed by the acid. The separated segment, when replaced in the main cast, fitted snugly like a piece in a jig-saw puzzle (*Fig.* 14).

This accidental finding was confirmed on another occasion by injecting the kidney in which one of the arteries entering the renal substance arose directly from the aorta, and had no connexion with the main stem of the renal artery. The main stem renal artery was injected with a red resin, and when this had set, the artery arising from the aorta was injected with a blue resin. When the cast was removed from the acid bath, it showed no transgression of colour between the bulk of the main cast and the smaller segment which fitted into it (*see Fig.* 9).

SECOND EXPERIMENT

As the previous injections had shown that the resin extended into the smallest vessels, and even filled the glomeruli, it seemed that the use of resins of a different colour might show if there was any seepage of colour between different segments. Two specimens were therefore injected so that each segment was filled with a resin of a different colour. This involved a rather delicate technique. A kidney with an arterial pattern of Group III was chosen in view of the easier arrangement of the vessels for access. A fine polythene cannula was introduced into the artery to the

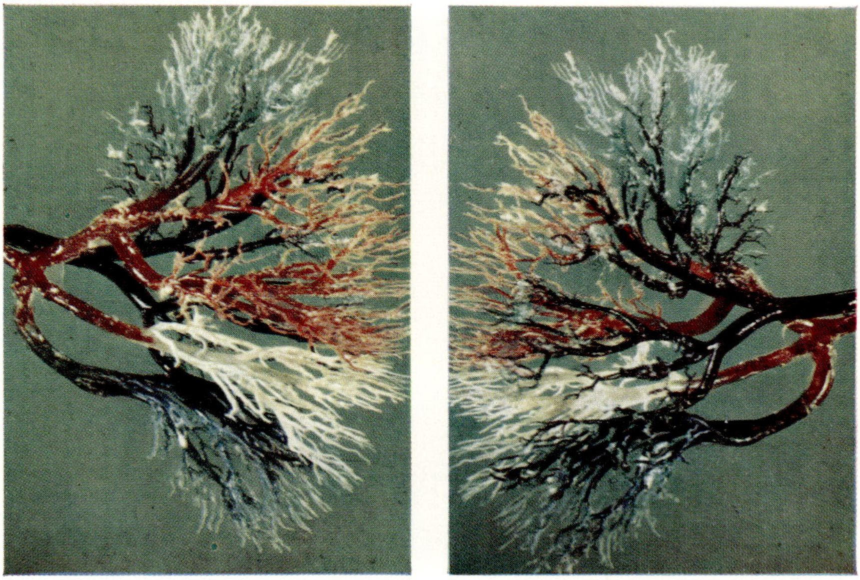

A B

FIG. 15.—A photograph in colour of a cast of the left kidney. A, The cast seen from the front. Each segment has been injected with a resin of a different colour. The apical segment is green, the upper segment red, the middle segment white, and the lower segment blue. B, The cast seen from behind. The posterior division and segment have been filled with black resin; the posterior branch of the lower segment artery is filled with blue resin. The arrangement of the anterior segment arteries is as in Group III.

apical segment through the lumen of the main renal artery. A quantity of green resin was injected, and a temporary ligature placed around the artery as soon as the polythene tube had been withdrawn, to avoid backflow of the resin. In the same manner the upper, middle, lower, and posterior segment arteries were each cannulated separately with a polythene tube and injected. The upper segment was injected with red, the middle segment with white, and the lower segment with blue resin (*Fig.* 15A). The posterior segment was injected with a black resin. In *Fig.* 15B the posterior branch of the lower segment artery, in blue resin, can be seen lying close to the black terminal branches of the posterior segment. Finally, when the resins in each segment had 'set', the temporary ligatures were removed and the remaining portions of the proximal portions of the segmental and main stem renal artery were filled with red resin, to produce a united cast.

Examination of the two casts, after removal from the acid bath, showed that there was a clear line of demarcation between each segment across which there was no transgression of colour from segment to segment.

Third Experiment

Although the two previous experiments had shown that there was no entry of resin from one segment to another, it was thought that this might still be possible, if the arteriolar pressure was greater in one segment than another. For example,

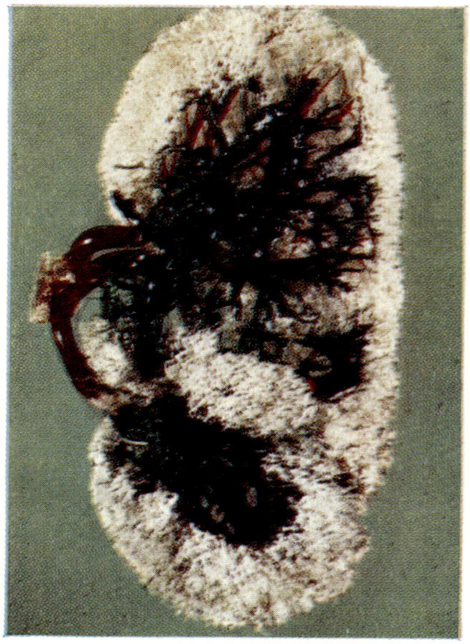

Fig. 16.—A photograph in colour of a cast of the left kidney, seen from the front. The venous system has been injected with green resin and the arteries with red resin. Prior to the arterial injection, the artery to the upper segment and a branch of the lower segment artery were ligated. The photograph shows the 'bare areas' corresponding to these ligations indicating that there is no collateral circulation from the surrounding segments.

arterial blood might pass to the upper and lower segments if the arterial pressure in these segments was lower than in the rest of the kidney. To put this question to the test, a kidney was taken, and its venous system injected with a green resin; the artery to the upper segment and part of the lower segment artery were then ligated at the hilum, so that no resin could enter their areas from the main renal artery. The latter was then injected with a red resin in the usual way. Subsequent examination of the cast (*Fig.* 16), showed that the areas corresponding to the ligated vessels were quite bare of the red arterial resin, so that the green resin of the underlying venous system was more easily visible.

The experiment was then repeated with more definition, this time being confined to the examination of one segment only—the middle segment. The artery to this segment was ligated first, and then the main renal artery injected with resin. The subsequent cast (*Fig.* 17) showed a 'bare area' corresponding to the middle segment.

The vessels visible in the lower part of the cast are the anterior and posterior branches of the lower segment artery, whilst those seen in the upper part of the 'bare area' are the branches of the upper segment artery and the terminal branches of the posterior segment artery seen behind.

It should be noted, however, that before any injection with resin was made into this particular kidney, it was subjected to a number of experiments with angiograms (as described in the next experiment), in order to try and obtain some correlation of facts produced by two different techniques.

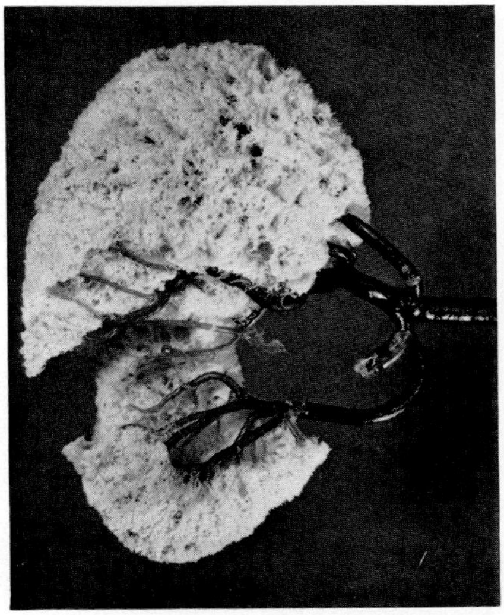

FIG. 17.—A cast of the right kidney (Group III) in which the artery to the middle segment was ligated before injection. The cast shows a 'bare area' corresponding to that segment. See *Fig*. 18E.

FOURTH EXPERIMENT

Although experience had so far shown that the resin penetrated the small arterioles and capillaries sufficiently well to show the glomerular tufts, it was thought that the molecular volume of the resin might be sufficiently large to prevent it passing along any small collateral channels which might exist between the segments. Further investigation was therefore necessary to exclude this.

Method of Investigation

A different method of investigation was necessary and radiography was selected on the grounds that arteriograms could be made, using radio-opaque materials of small molecular volume which would pass along any collateral channels which might exist.

TECHNIQUE OF RENAL ARTERIOGRAPHY

Post-mortem kidneys were perfused at a pressure approximating to that which they had received in life, and angiograms were made by the injection of 50 per cent and 70 per cent solutions of Diodone into the renal artery. At a later date when the angiograms had confirmed the absence of collateral circulation between the segments, a solution of sodium iodide was substituted for Diodone on account of the expense of the latter.

The renal vein was cannulated in order to lead away the drainage of the perfusate. Approximately 5–10 ml. Diodone were injected into the renal artery. The

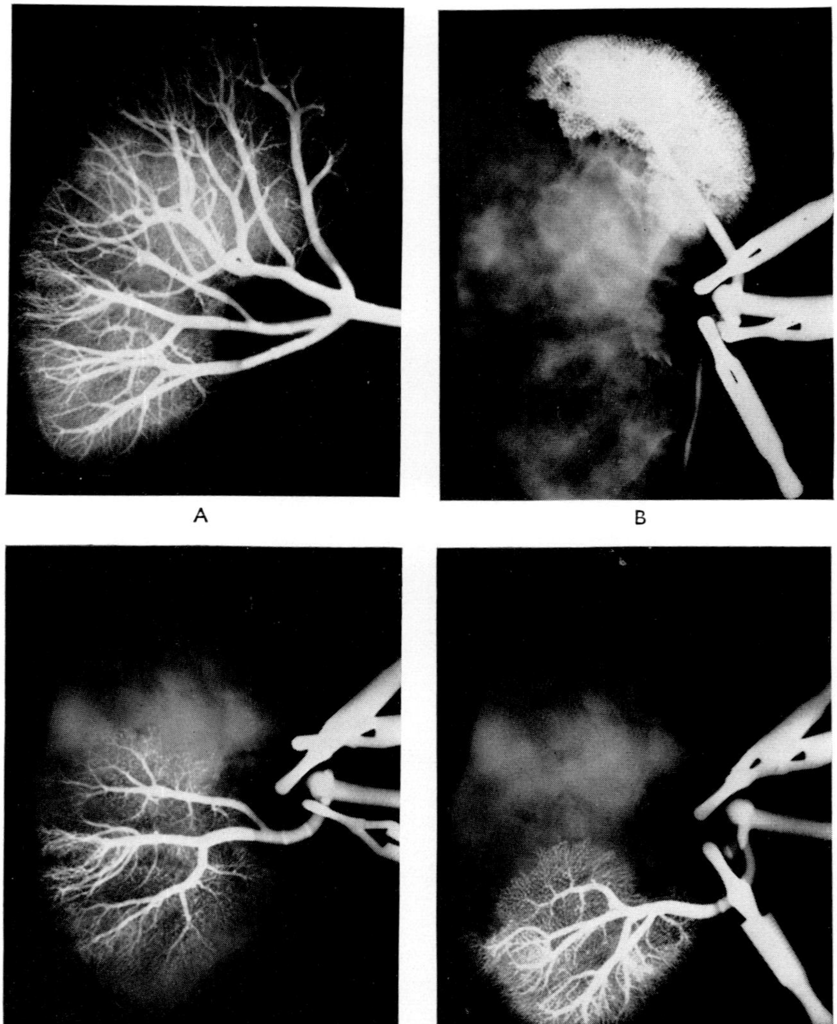

A B C D

FIG. 18.—An arteriogram of the same kidney as seen in *Fig.* 17. A, The complete arteriogram of the five segments. B, Arteriogram of the apical segment. The remaining segmental vessels have been occluded by clamps. C, Arteriogram of the middle segment. D, Arteriogram of the lower segment. Note the fine 'boutons' of the glomeruli. Compare this with E and also *Fig.* 17.

radiographic exposure was made at varying intervals after the injection, depending upon whether the main vessels or the segmental arterioles were to be visualized. Experimentation showed that an exposure of 0·8 second, at 45 kV. and 40 mA., the anode plate being 27 in. from the specimen, gave satisfactory pictures.

Difficulty was at first encountered in obtaining clear pictures. This was partly due to leakage of radio-opaque material from the small veins around the hilum and partly due to the lack of absorption of scattered X-rays.

A simple apparatus was made to overcome these problems. It consisted of a sheet of Perspex which was inclined at an angle of 60° to the horizontal plane upon which the kidney lay, so that the escaping perfusion fluid ran downwards away from the radiographic exposure field into a collecting trough below. The apparatus included a sliding device by which a radiographic film lying in contact with the under surface of the Perspex could be moved quickly under the specimen, thus enabling serial radiographs to be taken in rapid succession. The film was backed by sheet lead in the exposure chamber to absorb scattered X-rays and prevent halation.

Arteriograms were made of a number of kidneys, the first film in each case showing the distribution of the arteries throughout the whole organ (*Fig.* 18A). After the first injection had been made, the whole arterial system was flushed with perfusing fluid for a few minutes to remove any trace of radio-opaque material from the arteries and veins in order to give a clear field for the subsequent exposure. Occluding clamps were then applied to all the segmental arteries except one, and a second injection of Diodone and concurrent exposure made, thus producing a segmental arteriogram. After the exposure all the occluding clamps were removed,

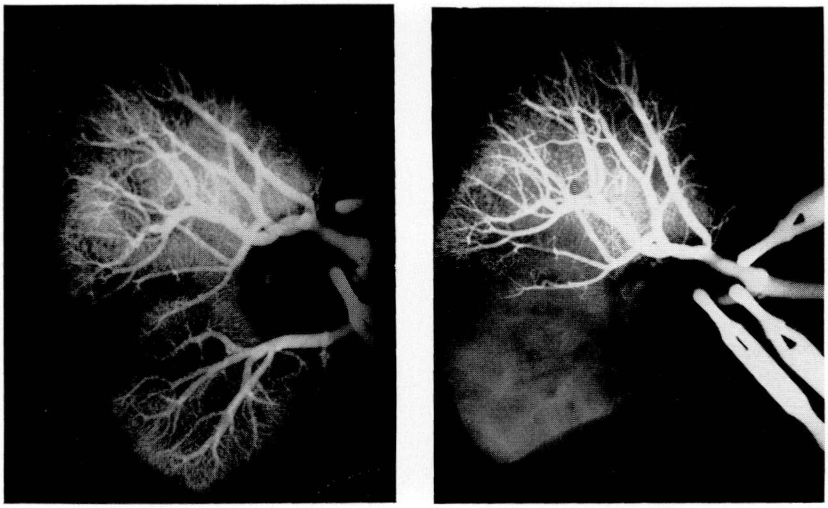

E F

FIG. 18 (*cont.*).—E, An arteriogram of all segments except the apical and middle segments which have been occluded. Compare this with *Fig.* 17; it shows clearly the area supplied by the posterior branch of the lower segment artery on the posterior aspect of the kidney. F, An arteriogram of the upper and posterior segments only.

the whole system flushed again, and the process was then repeated until arteriograms of all five segments had been obtained.

Results of Renal Arteriography

The investigation included sixty arteriograms on the human kidney. The intrarenal arteriography confirmed both the presence of a segmental arrangement and also that no collateral circulation existed between the arterial segments.

As shown in the segmental arteriograms *Fig.* 18B–F, the opaque dye has outlined only the segments concerned. *Fig.* 18B shows a segmental arteriogram of the apical segment; the area is well defined, the margins being clear cut. *Fig.* 18F shows a combined segmental arteriogram of the upper and posterior segments. The curve of the posterior segment artery is easily recognized as it sweeps across the

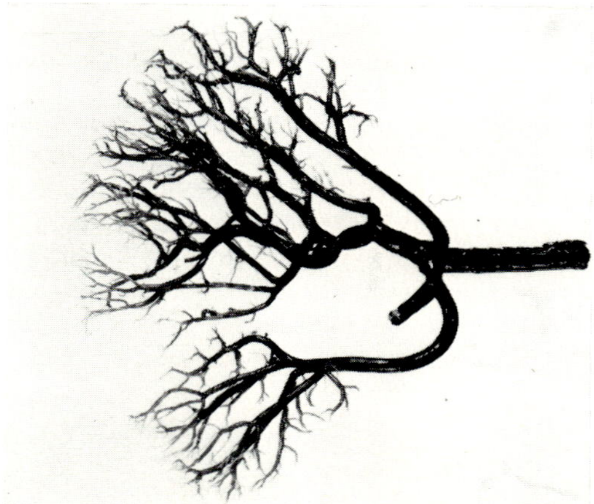

FIG. 19.—The same cast as shown in *Fig.* 17, after the cortical 'fluff' has been removed. Compare it with the arteriogram in *Fig.* 18E, to which it corresponds.

pelvis of the kidney. The middle and lower segments are outlined in *Fig.* 18 C and D. An analogous experiment to that of ligating the segmental artery to the middle segment prior to injection of resin was done, an arteriogram being made with an occlusion clamp on the artery to the middle segment and apical segment. *Fig.* 18E shows the 'bare area' of the middle segment corresponding to that on the cast as seen in *Figs.* 17 and 19.

Although it appears in *Fig.* 18E that the 'bare area' in the arteriogram is not so extensive as that in the cast, it is pointed out that the bridge of tissue in the middle of the 'bare area' of the arteriogram is formed by the adjacent borders of the posterior segment and the lower segment. The middle segment which has been excluded by the occlusion clamp is confined to the anterior surface of the kidney.

The complete arteriogram as shown in *Fig.* 18A can be reconstructed by the superimposition of the individual arteriograms. Similar segmental arteriograms are shown in *Fig.* 20.

This method of renal and segmental arteriography was of additional value in this investigation, since not only was the segmental pattern confirmed, but also by

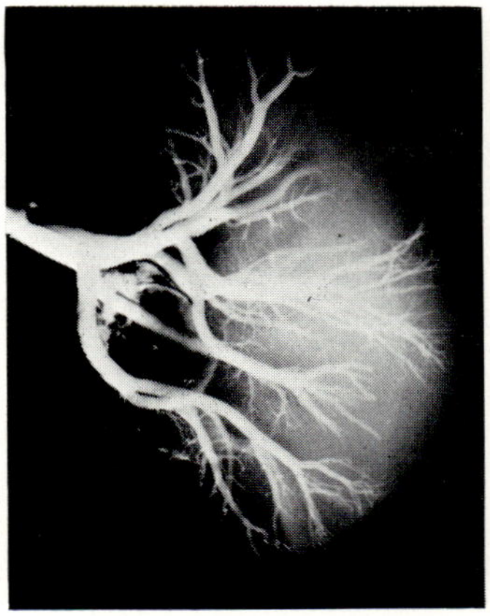

A

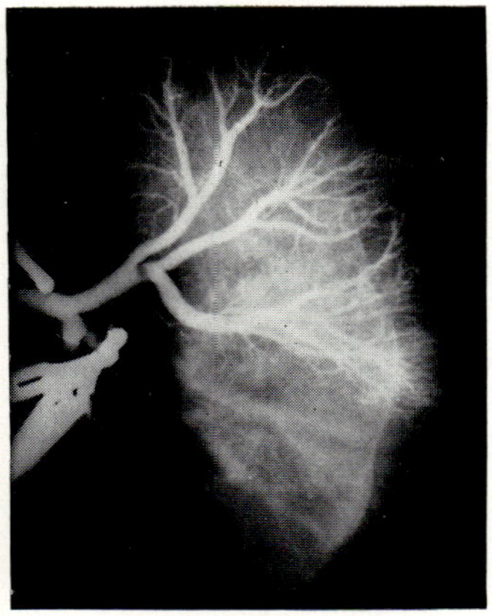

B

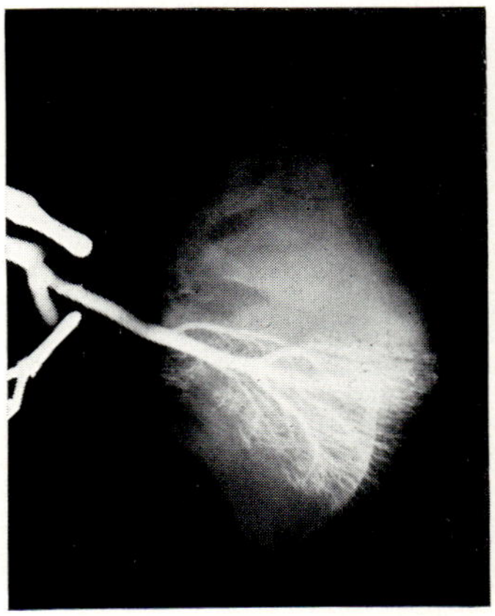

C

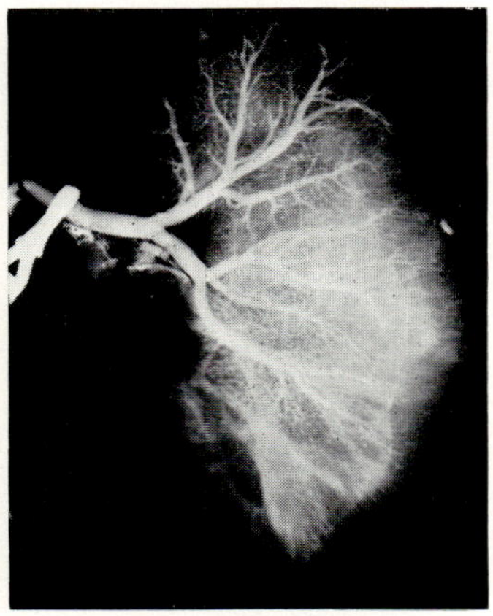

D

FIG. 20.—Arteriograms of the same kidney as shown in *Fig*. 15. A, The arteriogram of all the segments. B, Segmental arteriogram of the apical and upper segments. C, Segmental arteriogram of the middle segment. D, Segmental arteriogram of the posterior segment. E, Segmental arteriogram of the lower segment.

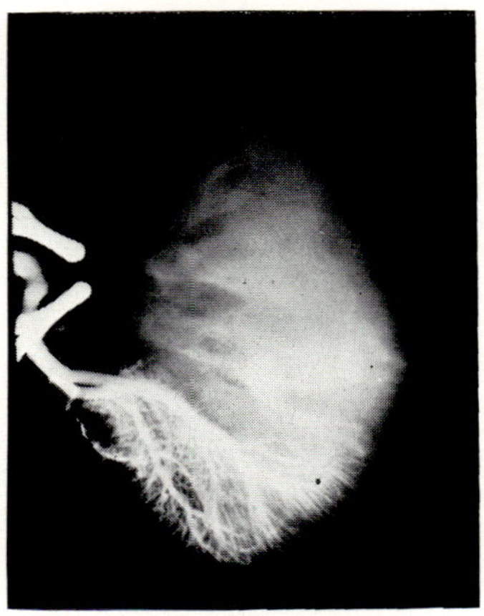

E

making arteriograms and segmental arteriograms of each specimen, and subsequently making a resin cast, comparison of the two enabled one to become conversant with the radiographic appearance of the renal arteriogram.

Further information has been given by examination of these arteriograms, especially those of *Fig.* 18C–E, in which the delicate pattern of the fine arterioles of the cortex, and even the 'boutons' of the glomerular tufts, can be recognized. The demonstration of this fine pattern is of particular importance as it is of value to know the appearance of these vessels in health, in order to appreciate their alteration in disease.

CHAPTER FOUR

THE INTRARENAL VEINS AND THE ABERRANT ARTERY

As the pattern and the nature of the intrarenal arterial system had now been determined, similar questions arose concerning that of the intrarenal venous system.

1. Is there a segmental pattern of the veins within the kidney, corresponding to that of the arteries?
2. Is there any communication between the intrarenal veins?

To seek an answer to these questions, similar methods were employed to those used in the investigations of the arterial system.

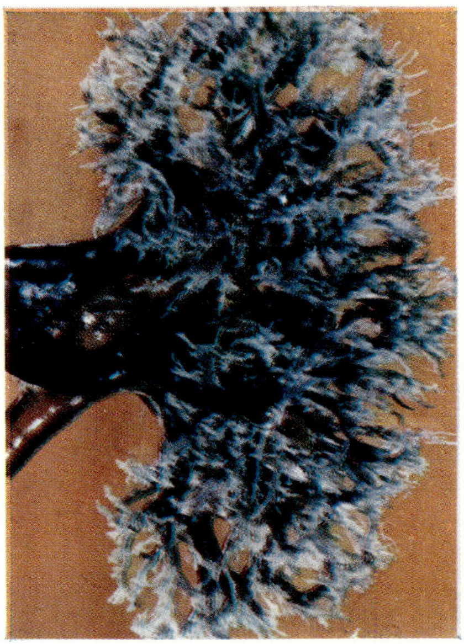

FIG. 21.—A cast of the venous system of the left kidney seen from the front. The entire system was filled by injection of one of the two main veins.

CASTS OF THE INTRARENAL VEINS

A post-mortem kidney was found which possessed three separate venous trunks at the hilum. A cannula was tied into the central vein and resin injected into it. Eventually the resin appeared at the mouths of the other two veins, indicating that there was, at any rate, an anastomosis at least between the major trunks.

Casts were then made of a number of kidneys, in which all the venous trunks leaving the kidney at the hilum were ligated, except one, which was retained patent for the purpose of injection. The intrarenal venous system only was injected, and to its full capacity, to examine the pattern of the communication between the veins. The resin cast showed to perfection the shape and form of the kidney and was, if anything, more beautiful in its sponge-like appearance than the cast produced by injection of the arterial system. It had also a very definite difference in the finer texture in the capillary venules of the cortex, in that these lay in palisades at right-angles to the surface of the kidney. Also, in contrast to the arterial casts, and as one might expect, the resin did not enter and produce the tiny 'bouton' casts of the glomerular tufts.

A study of the larger venous channels within the kidney showed that the main venous trunks which enter the hilum vary from one to four. Within the substance of the kidney these trunks divide into smaller branches, between which connecting channels pass (*Fig.* 21). These are most evident in the cortex of the kidney where the smaller veins form a series of arcades lying mainly in the longitudinal axis of the kidney (*Fig.* 22). There are usually three systems of longitudinal arcades, in parallel planes, and smaller arcades link those of different planes with one another.

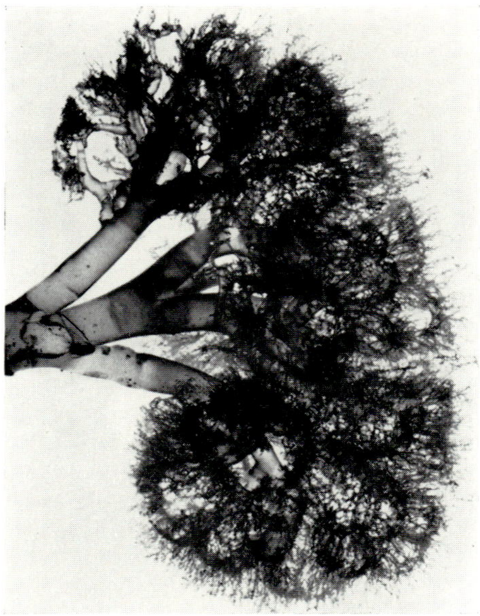

FIG. 22.—A cast of the intrarenal venous system, photographed by transmitted light. This shows at least three of the parallel systems of arcades which run mainly in the longitudinal axis of the kidney, giving a free anastomosis.

ANGIOGRAPHY OF THE INTRARENAL VEINS

The same facts were found concerning the veins on perfusing the venous system with water or saline, for irrigation of one main venous trunk produced an equivalent flow of fluid from the other vein. Similarly radiographic angiography of the intrarenal veins produced the same evidence as did examination of the casts.

In conclusion it has been shown by these studies that, in contrast to the intrarenal arteries, the intrarenal veins present no segmental arrangement at all, there being a free anastomosis of the venous channels throughout the kidney. This confirms the findings of John Hunter of 1794, and more recently of Lee Brown in 1924.

'THE ARCUATE ARTERIES OF THE KIDNEY'—A POSSIBLE EXPLANATION

As already mentioned in an earlier chapter, some of the older anatomical texts make mention of 'arcuate' or 'arciform' arteries of the kidney, and imply that there is a free anastomosis of arterial blood through the lumen of these vessels. So far, my own investigations have shown no existence of such an arterial anastomosis—in fact have shown precisely to the contrary. There is, I suggest, a possible explanation for these 'arcuate vessels' which were previously described.

If a post-mortem kidney is taken and a cast made of the pelvi-caliceal system with a red resin and the venous system with a clear resin, it will be seen that there is a considerable plexus of fine veins around each calix, and also the necks of the calices.

A second kidney is now taken and injected as before with the same coloured resins—red for the pelvi-calicine and clear resin for the venous system. On this occasion, however, the pelvi-calicine system is injected *first, with some pressure, and before the venous system has been filled with resin.* When the subsequent cast is examined, it will be found, not infrequently, that some of the red resin from the pelvi-calicine system has ruptured into the fine veins which lie around it, with the result that the clear resin of the venous system contains streaks of red, often extending far into the venous arcades.

Now this occurrence is probably by the same mechanism as that encountered in clinical radiography, in which 'pyelovenous back-flow' is seen in retrograde pyelograms, when the opaque dye injected up the ureteric catheter extravasates beyond the limits of the pelvi-calicine collecting system.

I suggest, therefore, that the 'arcuate' or 'arciform' arteries are probably artifacts, produced perhaps by ruptures into the veins due to the high pressure necessary when injecting, in byegone days, such tenacious mixtures as red lead and gelatine.

THE ABERRANT RENAL ARTERY

Aberrant or accessory renal arteries have been of interest to the clinician for many years, mainly because of the possible part that the vessel may play in the causation of hydronephrosis. Many cases have been described in the literature in which an aberrant or accessory artery is found to enter the lower pole of the kidney, and to lie in such a position as to appear to obstruct the outflow of the urine at the pelvi-ureteric junction.

Schools of thought are divided as to whether the obstruction is, in fact, due to kinking of the ureter by the vessel, or whether it is due to a so-far unexplained neuromuscular incoordination at the pelvi-ureteric junction. Opinion is also divided on the advisability of dividing the aberrant vessel, both as to the effects that this may have upon the obstruction, and on the possibility of resultant necrosis of part of the kidney.

Hitherto a widely held view has been that normally the kidney is supplied by a single renal artery which enters the hilum and that any additional artery entering the kidney at one or other pole is necessarily an extra and aberrant source of supply to that provided by the main stem of the renal artery. Such vessels entering the upper pole of the kidney arise from either the aorta or the suprarenal artery, whereas those entering the lower pole may stem from the aorta, common or internal iliac vessels and even the superior mesenteric artery (Anson, Cauldwell, Pick, and Beaton, 1948).

Georges Gerard in 1911, in his study of 150 pairs of kidneys, was probably the first to recognize that the presence of additional vessels at the hilum was due to an early division of the main renal artery, rather than a true multiplication or increase in the number of arteries. He did not, however, study the vessels within the kidney substance in conjunction with those of the pedicle, his conclusions being based on the study of the pedicle alone.

This concept is important, not only for the understanding of the arterial pattern in the study of anatomy, but also for the practice of surgery, since the ligation of a vessel on the grounds that it is an accessory artery will lead to necrosis of a segment or part of a segment.

In his original diagram (*Fig.* 23), Gerard commented that the number of branches at the hilum was greater when the renal artery had undergone precocious division.

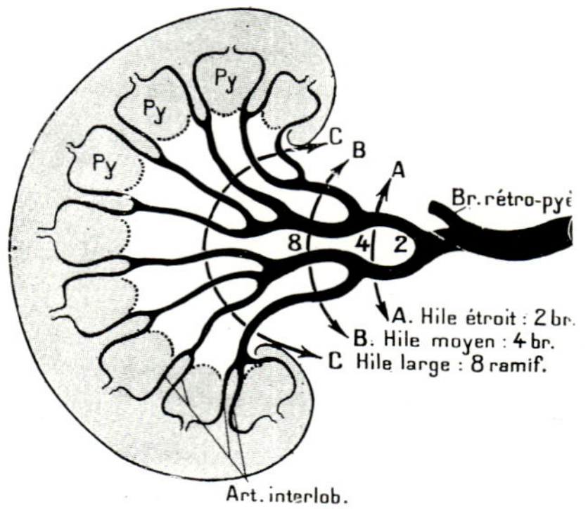

FIG. 23.—A diagram made by Gerard (1911), indicating his conception of the method of division of the anterior branches of the renal artery depending upon the size of the hilum of the kidney. The hilum at A was small, whilst that at C represented a large hilum.

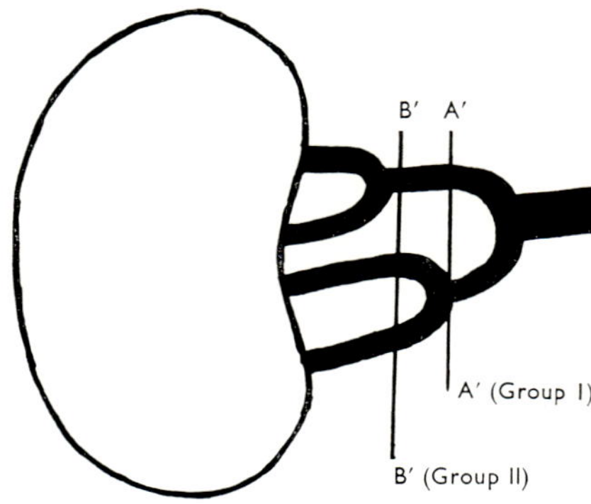

FIG. 24.—An interesting academic point showing that if Gerard had drawn the lines A–A and B–B, more obliquely, as in this diagram of mine, then the figure would represent the arrangement of the middle and lower segment arteries of Group I and Group II respectively.

This division was not dichotomous and concerned only the anterior branches of the main artery. The number of branches of the anterior division would be two, with the hilum at positions A—A, and four in the case of an earlier division of the main stem, at position B—B. My own investigation shows an interesting, although perhaps rather academic point, that if the lines drawn by Gerard had been made rather more oblique, as in my modifications of A′—A′ and B′—B′ (*Fig.* 24), then the picture represents, in diagrammatic form, the arrangement of the middle and lower segment arteries of Group I and Group II which I have already described.

The incidence of aberrant arteries has been variously reported as nearly 50 per cent (Hellström, 1927) and 25 per cent (Edsman, 1954). A number of authors have recorded that in cases where more than one renal artery is present, those to the lower pole are the most frequent. Weinstein, Countiss, and Derbes (1940) found that the incidence of 'accessory' vessels passing from the aorta to the lower pole was approximately twice that of those going to the upper pole. The same fact is recorded by Albarran (1909).

In my first series it was found that in 63 per cent of casts the lower segment artery had the most proximal origin of the three segmental arteries in the anterior division, for it may arise from the anterior division, or at any point along the main renal artery, or indeed directly from the aorta itself.

Judging by the many descriptions of these vessels in the literature, it is evident that there is no established criterion for aberrance; the term has been applied equally to an additional artery in the renal pedicle, or to a vessel entering the kidney at either pole, whether derived from the main renal artery, from the aorta, or from a branch of the aorta.

In order to clarify the situation, from the viewpoints of both the anatomist and the surgeon, it is necessary to consider two questions:—

First, what contribution do accessory or aberrant arteries make to the blood-supply of the kidney? The answer to this is clear. Study of the series of casts described in previous chapters has shown that if the arteries of the renal pedicle are examined in conjunction with those within the kidney substance, and not regarded as a separate entity, as is so often the case in standard teaching of anatomy and surgery, then it becomes obvious that the so-called 'aberrant' and 'accessory' arteries are not so, for they are *normal segmental arteries with a precocious origin*, and whose blood-flow is in no way an extra supply to that of the main stem (*see Figs.* 9, 10, pp. 11, 12).

Secondly, *how can the presence of aberrant vessels, and their range of pattern, be explained*? The answer to this question is somewhat more complex, for it involves the study not only of the single 'aberrant' vessel, but also the wider range of multiple renal vessels, and indeed of the whole arterial pattern of the congenitally abnormal kidney.

This is described in the next chapter.

CHAPTER FIVE

THE CONGENITALLY ABNORMAL KIDNEY

So far, investigations into the renal vascular anatomy have been confined to the normal kidney. There remained a small, but none the less distinct group, in which no investigations had yet been done—that is, those in which the kidney is congenitally abnormal. As the latter are equally (and in some surgeons' view, more likely) to be affected by disease processes as their normal fellows, a study of their arterial anatomy was obviously necessary, for conservation of renal tissue is equally important to the patient with a horse-shoe kidney as to his more fortunate brother.

This chapter reports the work of the past sixteen years, in which congenitally abnormal kidneys have been collected for investigation from the London area and the Midlands. By the very nature of their rarity, it will be appreciated that the series is small in comparison with the original work on normal kidneys.

MATERIAL AND METHODS OF INVESTIGATION

This investigation has involved the study of some 37 casts of kidneys whose position or form was unusual, or whose blood-supply appeared to be different from that usually found. The series included the examination of 11 'horse-shoe' and 1 pelvic, ectopic kidney. Additional facts were culled from clinical aortograms and findings at operation.

The major part of the work was carried out on post-mortem specimens. These were obtained by the courtesy of a number of pathologists from a very wide area.

In order to study the arterial vessels which might have connexion in any way with the renal substance, a very extensive portion of retroperitoneal tissue had to be obtained. It was important that this tissue should be removed in one piece, for any dissection in the area might destroy the very evidence which was sought. The excised tissue extended from the diaphragm to the junction of the internal and external iliac vessels, and included the aorta, both kidneys, adrenals, and the neighbouring fat and vessels. The aorta was then closed at one end and the whole specimen irrigated with saline or water to remove remaining blood-clot.

In suitable cases arteriograms were first carried out, and when these had been completed, a resin cast of the specimen was made. A similar technique to that previously described was used. A liquid polyester resin (Marco Resin, S.B.61c) was mixed with a monomer and catalyst, and then injected into the aorta. Within a few minutes, as a result of the chemical action, the liquid resin became solid, and 'set' in the shape of the arteries in which it lay. The whole specimen was then placed in a bath of concentrated hydrochloric acid, which removed the organic tissue by the process of corrosion, leaving the resin cast untouched.

ARTERIAL SEGMENTS OF THE NORMAL KIDNEY

In order to appreciate the significance of the arterial anatomy in the congenitally abnormal kidney, it is necessary to have some knowledge of that found in the normal organ. This has been described in earlier chapters, and is given here only in brief, for convenience, and to remind the reader of the essential facts.

The distribution of the arteries within the kidney substance is constant and upon this is founded the division of the renal parenchyma into five segments. These have been named the apical, upper, middle, lower, and posterior segments. The middle and upper segments lie in the anterior plane of the kidney, whilst the posterior lies in the posterior plane. The apical and lower segments, however, differ from the remainder in that they occupy areas in both anterior and posterior planes. The main stem of the renal artery divides at any point between the aorta and the hilum into an anterior and posterior division. The latter continues to supply the posterior segment, whereas the former supplies the upper, middle, and lower segments, and frequently the apical as well.

Arrangement of the Segmental Arteries

The Apical Artery

This is very variable in its origin, but most commonly stems from the anterior division, or the artery to the upper segment. Less commonly it arises from the posterior division, and on occasions makes an extrahilar entry (Type III), having arisen from the aorta itself. The variations of this Type III will be described later.

The Upper Segment Artery

On entry into the kidney substance it divides into an apical branch, and a lateral or horizontal branch.

The Middle Segment Artery

It also arises from the anterior division. If the upper and lower calices are large, and there are no middle calices, then the middle segment and its artery are correspondingly small. This fact, first noted in 1953, has subsequently been found to have its counterpart in some 'horse-shoe' kidneys.

The Lower Segment Artery

This also is a branch of the anterior division. Soon after entering its segment, it divides into an anterior branch which passes in front of the calix, and a posterior branch which runs under the neck of the lower calix and supplies the posterior aspect of the lower pole. *It is of importance to appreciate the existence of this posterior branch, for it also has its counterpart in renal anomalies.* The lower segment artery is perhaps the most interesting of all the segmental arteries for, whilst conforming to the law in the area it supplies, its method of doing so is very varied. These variations themselves, however, still follow an ordered pattern, which becomes the more obvious as the anomalous kidneys are studied.

THE ARTERIAL SUPPLY OF THE CONGENITALLY ABNORMAL KIDNEY

The investigation was carried out on four groups of renal abnormality:—

A. The kidney whose pelvi-calicine system was abnormal (e.g., 'duplex kidney').

B. The kidney whose substance was normal, but whose arterial supply consisted of more than the single, statutory renal artery.

C. The kidney whose substance and site was abnormal (e.g., 'horse-shoe kidney').

D. The kidney whose site was abnormal.

The work was designed to seek an answer to the following questions:—

a. Is it possible to recognize an arterial pattern in so widely diverse a series of anomalies, and is there any relation to the normal?

b. If arterial segments do exist in renal anomalies, is there any collateral circulation between them?

c. Lastly, can any explanation be found for such arterial variations?

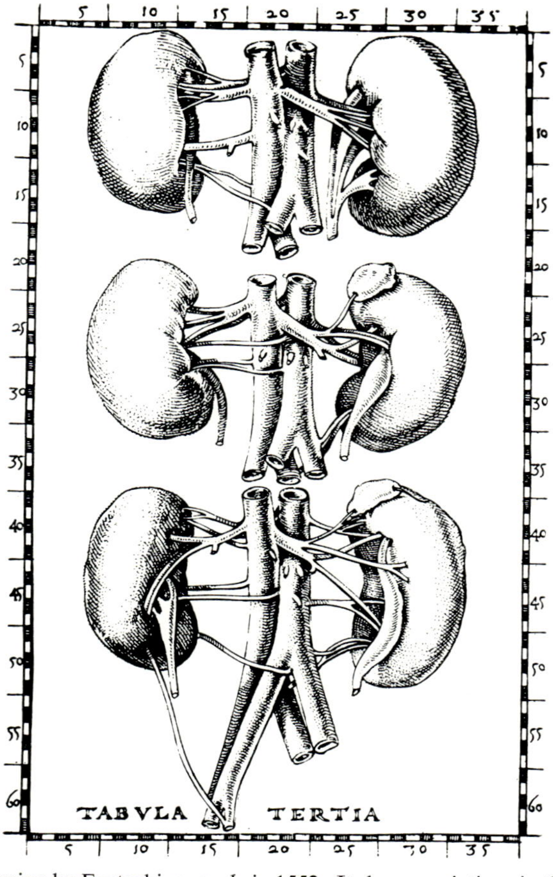

FIG. 25.—A drawing by Eustachius, made in 1552. It shows variations in the arterial supply to the kidney, particularly of vessels entering the lower pole. These arise, severally, from the common iliac, the aorta, the bifurcation of the aorta, and also the internal iliac artery.

A. THE KIDNEY WITH ABNORMAL PELVI-CALICINE SYSTEM

Ten casts were examined of kidneys in which the pelvis was either bifid, or in which two separate pelves and separate ureters existed. No very significant variation of the arterial pattern was found, other than those already described in normal kidneys. Unfortunately, no specimen could be obtained of a kidney in which the renal substance itself lay in two separate parts. I have, however, gained an overall impression that the arteries are relatively little affected by the behaviour of the pelvi-calicine system, apart from the fact already mentioned that the size of the segmental vessels may be smaller in those areas where the calices are smaller.

B. The Kidney with Multiple Renal Arteries

It is of some historical interest that in 1552 such anomalous or aberrant arteries were recorded by Eustachius, who illustrated amongst others three kidneys (*Fig.* 25), in which arteries entering the lower half of the kidney arose respectively from the aorta, the common iliac, and the internal iliac arteries. These plates were drawn by

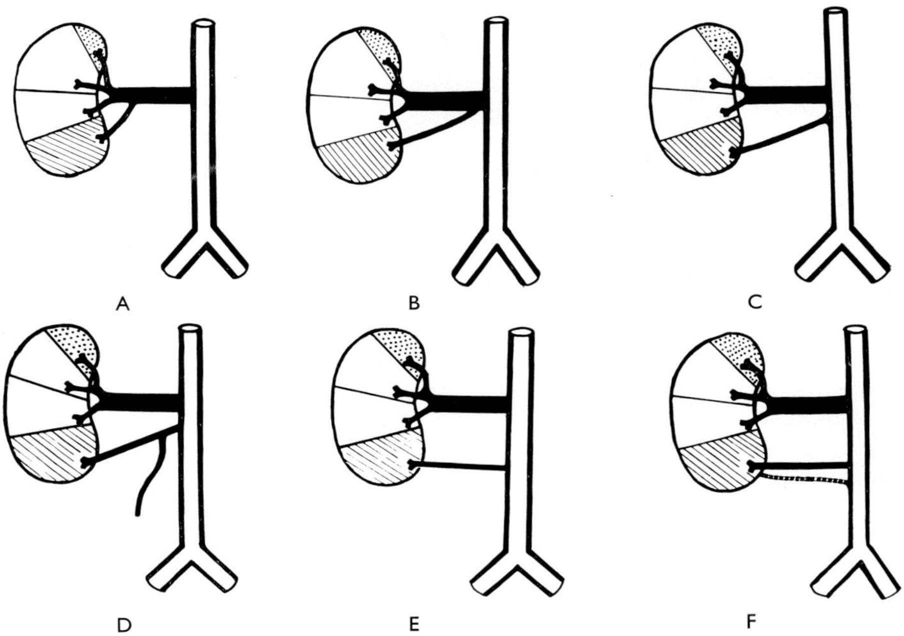

FIG. 26.—A diagram illustrating the variations of origin of the artery to the lower segment of the kidney. The artery arises: A, At the hilum; B, From the main stem at its junction with the aorta; C, From the aorta close to the main stem; D, From the aorta but also giving rise to the testicular or ovarian artery. E, The lower segment artery arises from the aorta at some distance from the main stem. F, The lower segment artery and its posterior branch arise separately from the aorta.

Eustachius himself. They remained unprinted and were stored in the Papal Library for 162 years, until eventually Pope Clement XI found, and presented the engraved plates to his Physician, Lancisi, who, upon the advice of Morgagni, published them with his own notes in 1714.

In a previous paragraph I showed that although the renal segments and their arteries are constantly present, their origins from the renal artery have some variation, and that the point of division may not always be confined to the hilum.

These variations were classified into groups. It was found that the apical and lower segment arteries, on occasions, not only arose from the renal artery quite independently from the remainder of the segmental vessels, but also frequently did so directly from the aorta itself. Perhaps the most important contribution to our knowledge was that study of these vessels by casts and arteriograms showed that these so-called 'extra' or 'aberrant and anomalous' arteries were in no degree 'extra'. They were, in fact, normal segmental vessels whose origin was more

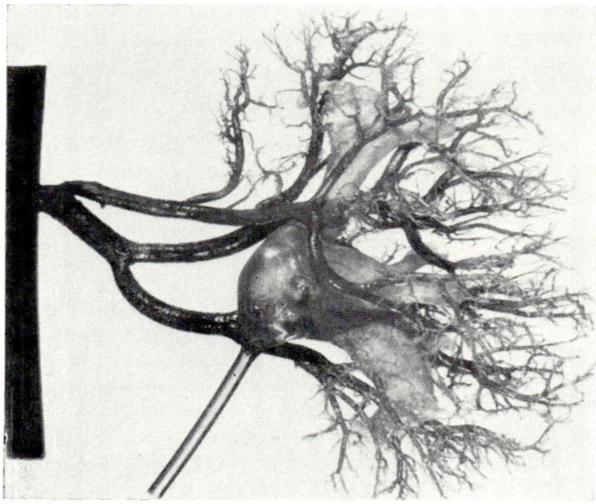

FIG. 27.—A cast of the right kidney seen from behind. This shows an unusually proximal origin of the anterior and posterior divisions. The main stem is only $\frac{1}{4}$ in. long.

proximal than usual, and that ligation or division of them would result in ischaemia of the segment of renal tissue which they supplied.

In recent years further specimens have been examined and classified. It is hoped that this study will not only provide some knowledge of assistance in operative surgery, but will also, in conjunction with the study of embryology, throw some light on the reason why these arterial variations occur.

The variations of the segmental arteries to the kidney, appearing as aberrant or multiple vessels, can be classified into three groups: (1) At the hilum; (2) In the pedicle; (3) From the aorta.

1. Variations at the Hilum

The artery to the lower segment is the only vessel originating at the hilum whose course may appear unusual, for sometimes it is long and winding (Group II: *Fig.* 26A).

2. Variations in the Pedicle

The presence of more than one artery in the pedicle may be due to:—

a. Early division of the main stem at a point close to the aorta, into anterior and posterior divisions, thus giving the impression of two renal arteries (*Fig.* 27).

b. The apical segment artery arising from the junction of the main stem with the aorta, as in Type IIIa (*Fig.* 28).

c. The lower segment artery arising close to, or from, the junction of the main stem with the aorta (*Fig*. 26B).

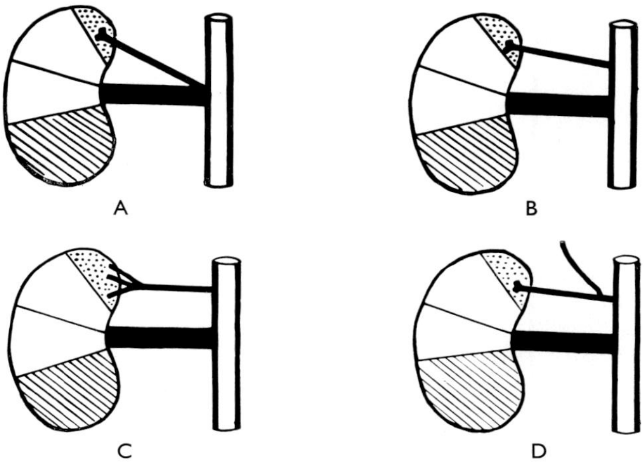

FIG. 28.—A diagram of the variations of Type III of the artery to the apical segment. The artery arises: A, From the main stem close to the aorta; B, From the aorta; C, From the aorta but dividing into a leash of vessels each of which enters the segment separately; D, From the aorta, the suprarenal artery arising from it.

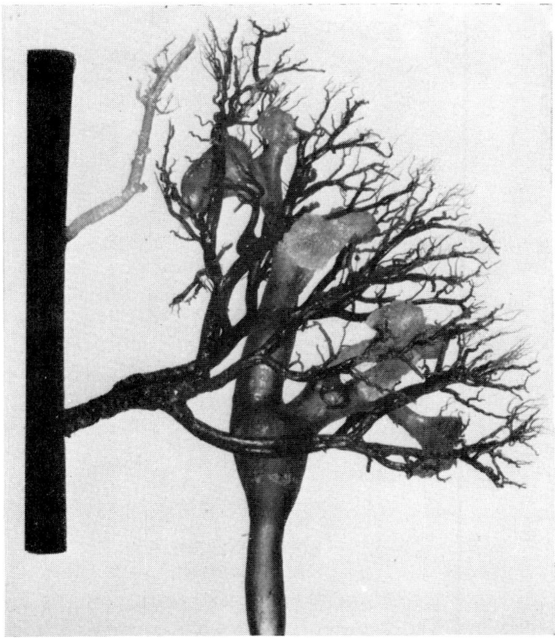

FIG. 29.—A cast of the left kidney seen from the front. The apical segment artery, outlined in pale resin, arises directly from the aorta at some distance from the main stem.

3. Variations from the Aorta

The most common arrangement in this group is that of a single artery arising from the aorta together with a normal renal artery, the artery to the lower segment being the most frequent example. The arteries which can arise directly from the aorta are:—

a. The anterior and posterior divisions (*see Fig.* 27).

b. The artery to the apical segment.

These are variants of Type III (*see Fig.* 28). The artery may arise from the aorta (*Fig.* 29) above that of the main stem, and enter its segment at once (Type IIIb; *see Fig.* 28), or may break into a leash of vessels each of which enters the

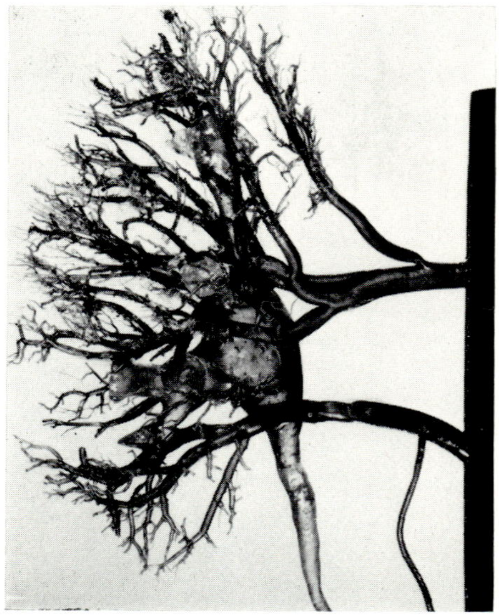

FIG. 30.—A cast of the right kidney seen from the front. The apical segment artery arises from the main stem (Type IIIa), the lower segment artery arises from the aorta; it is a large vessel and gives origin to the artery to the testicle or ovary.

segment separately (Type IIIc). It may alternatively arise jointly with or from the adrenal artery (Type IIId).

c. Artery to the lower segment. It is impossible to list all the slight differences of origin of this vessel. In the main, however, they fall into these groups:—

i. It may arise direct from the aorta, at a point a little below that of the main stem (*see Fig.* 26C).

ii. It may arise direct from the aorta, but also give origin to the testicular or ovarian artery (*see Figs.* 26D, 30).

iii. It may arise at a much lower level (*see Fig.* 26E).

iv. As in the previous case it may arise low down from the aorta, but instead of dividing into anterior and posterior branches within the renal substance, these two branches arise directly and independently from the aorta (*see Figs.* 26F, 31).

There is, in fact, no real difference between the variations of the so-called 'normal' kidney and those of the apparently grossly abnormal kidney with four 'aberrant' renal arteries. *Table I* summarizes the situation, for clarity and convenience.

Table I.—DIFFERENT COMBINATIONS OF ARTERIES APPEARING AS 'ABERRANT VESSELS'

ARTERY	VARIATIONS IN THE 'NORMAL' (DIVISION AT THE HILUM)	VARIATIONS PRESENTING AS 'ABERRANTS'		
		At the Hilum	In the Pedicle	From the Aorta
Main stem	—	—	Early origin of divisions	Separate origin of divisions
Apical segment	Types I, II, and IV	—	Type IIIa	Types IIIb, c, and d
Lower segment	Type A arranged with other anterior segment arteries as in Groups I, II, and III	Group I with long lower segment artery	Type B	Types C, D, E, and F

The Kidney with Four Renal Arteries

Of these I have only two cases—one being an arterial cast, and one a clinical arteriogram. This anomaly is of particular interest, not only because of its rarity, but also because *it provides a link with our knowledge of embryology, and with the arterial supply of the horse-shoe kidney.* Four arteries were found to enter the kidney from the aorta and each was injected separately with a resin of different colour. The patch of pink resin in the midst of paler and diluted yellow and blue resins illustrates, as in normal kidneys, that there is no collateral circulation between one arterial segment and another (*Fig.* 31). The four vessels, from above downwards, are:— The posterior division (yellow resin); the anterior division (red resin), supplying the upper and middle segments; below this, the anterior branch of the lower segment (blue resin); and lastly, the posterior branch of the lower segment artery (red resin). The artery to the apical segment arises from the posterior division, being of Type IV.

Embryology of the Renal Arteries

The proximal origin of the segmental arteries of the kidney can be explained by reference to the account of the development of the mesonephric arteries by Felix (1912).

The mesonephric arteries develop on each side of the aorta, being distributed throughout the mesonephric area, from the sixth cervical to the third lumbar segments. At first they supply the mesonephros only, but later they supply, in addition, the suprarenal glands, the renal or metanephric mass, and also the reproductive glands. As growth occurs, the more cranial part of the mesonephros, together with its vessels, disappears before those at the caudal end have reached their maximal development. The mesonephric arteries in the thoracolumbar region traverse an area which is occupied in varying degrees at different levels by the suprarenal gland, the mesonephros laterally, and more ventrally the reproductive gland. Within this area the arteries form a network, the *rete arteriosum*

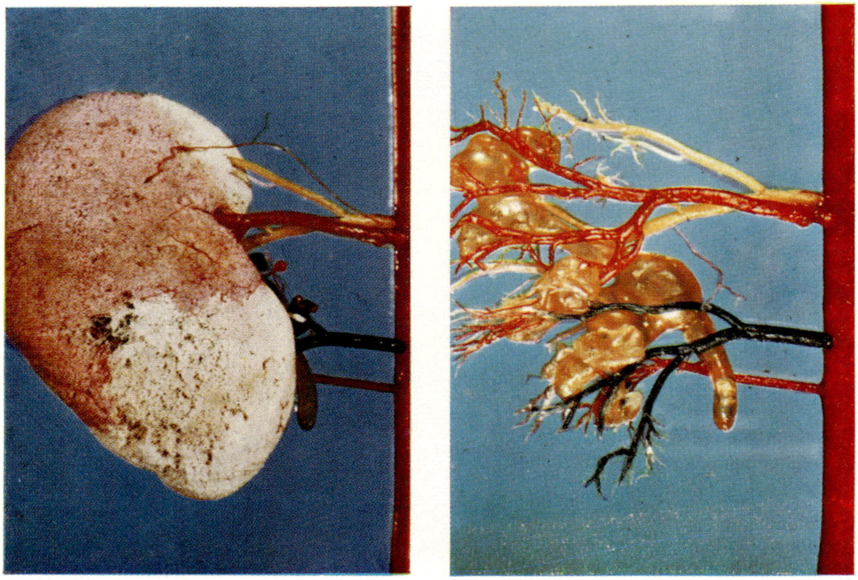

A B

FIG. 31.—A, A colour photograph of a cast of the right kidney seen from the front. From above downwards the yellow vessels are the apical segment artery and the posterior division. The anterior division is injected with red resin. Below this is the anterior branch of the lower segment artery in blue resin, and lastly, the posterior branch of the lower segment artery in red resin. B, The same cast as in A, after the 'fluff' produced by the resin in the glomeruli has been removed. This shows the segmental arteries well. Note the similarity of this photograph to the diagram of the mesonephric arteries in *Fig.* 32B.

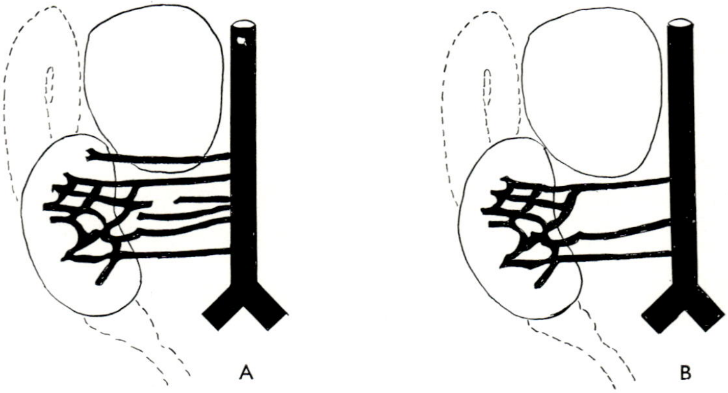

A B

FIG. 32.—A, A diagram after Felix, showing the mesonephric arteries, some of which are degenerating, leaving the rete arteriosum urogenitale to be supplied by the neighbouring roots. B, In my modification of this diagram these degenerating roots have been removed to illustrate the similarity to the cast in *Fig.* 31B.

urogenitale. From this network the mesonephros, metanephros, and the gonads are supplied with arterial vessels, these organs thus being independent of single branches for their blood-supply. Eventually some of the roots which supply this network degenerate, the area which they previously supplied being taken over by a neighbouring root. In the diagram after Felix (*Fig*. 32A), there are shown the mesonephric arteries, some of which are degenerating. In my adjacent modification of this diagram (*Fig*. 32B) the degenerating arteries have been removed. Comparison of this diagram with the photograph of the arterial cast (*Fig*. 31B) presents a startling similarity which strongly suggests that the persistence of some mesonephric arteries could account for the variation of origin of the adult segmental arteries from the aorta.

One other explanation can perhaps be supplied by embryology. It has been noted that of all the segmental arteries of the adult kidney, that to the lower segment is the most frequent in having a direct origin from the aorta. I suggest that this may be explained by the fact that the caudal mesonephric arteries, being the last to form, are the least likely to be affected by the degenerative processes which have already been carried out on the more cranial mesonephric vessels.

C. The 'Horse-shoe' Kidney

Casts were made of 13 'horse-shoe' kidneys, including 1 from a baby. The specimens were obtained post mortem.

The Nature of the Blood-supply

In a number of cases, arteriograms were made for comparison with the casts, and also on occasions casts were made by multiple resin injection; that is to say, different arteries were cannulated separately through the aorta and injected with different coloured resins. Both these experiments confirmed, as in normal kidneys, that each artery supplied its own area, and that there is no collateral circulation between these areas.

The Arrangement of the Arteries

Study of the casts showed that, in general, the 'horse-shoe' kidney can be regarded, as far as the arteries are concerned, as two separate kidneys, which either approximate or are continuous across the midline. This is particularly true of the arteries to the upper, middle, and posterior segments, which show little variation from the normal. These vessels arise from the aorta at the normal level, but tend to angulate downwards, for in most 'horse-shoe' kidneys the cortical substance of the kidney lies much lower than usual. This may be due to medial rotation. Although there were considerable small variations in the arterial pattern, on the whole the arrangement of the blood-supply tended to fall into fairly definite groups. These were:—

Type H-S I

Only one specimen was found in this group, which was that of a pair of kidneys, approximating but not actually fused, in the midline. Each kidney was supplied by a single artery, whose segmental vessels tended to divide early in the pedicle, and which corresponded to Group I on one side and Group II on the other (*Fig*. 33).

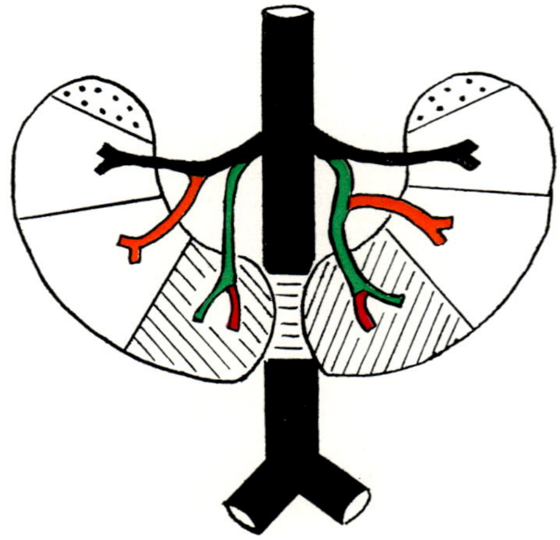

FIG. 33.—A diagram illustrating the first variation of blood-supply to the horse-shoe kidney. Type H-S I shows two kidneys approximated but not joined across the midline. The arrangement of the arterial pattern is that of two normal kidneys, i.e., Group I and Group II. The arteries to the upper, middle, and lower segments have been coloured, black, orange, and green respectively. The branch of the lower segment artery which has been coloured red, indicates the posterior branch of that vessel.

TYPE H-S IIa

The segmental arteries to the apical, upper, middle, and posterior segments on both sides of the midline are as in a normal kidney. The arteries of the lower segment follow their mesonephric tendency to arise direct from the aorta on either side. Once within the renal substance, however, they divide as usual into branches which correspond to the anterior and posterior branches of the normal kidney (*Figs*. 34, 35).

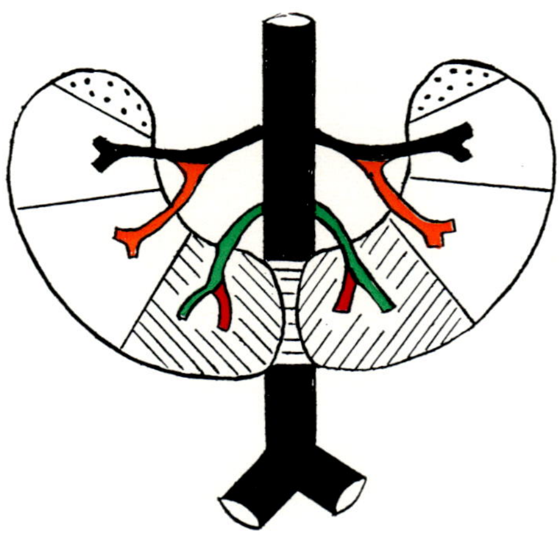

FIG. 34.—Type H-S IIa; similar to H-S I, but both lower segment arteries arise independently from the aorta. The colour scheme is standardized to that of *Fig*. 33.

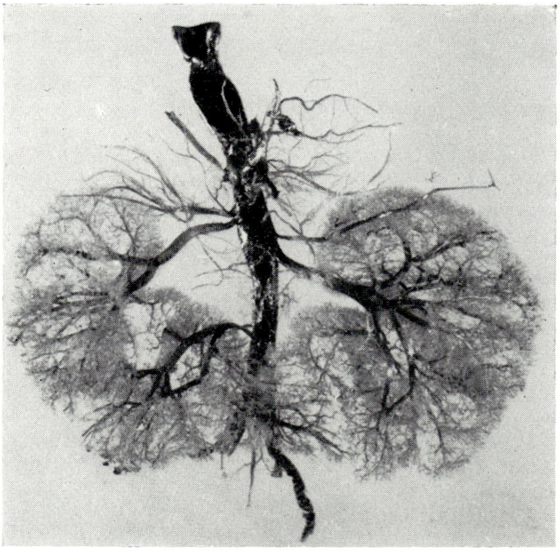

FIG. 35.—A cast of a horse-shoe kidney of a baby. The kidneys are in contact across the midline. The left kidney is that of a normal kidney with a single main stem artery; the right kidney is that of Type H-S IIa, in which the lower segment artery arises independently from the aorta.

TYPE H-S IIb

A variation of the above, but is perhaps more common. The arterial arrangement is the same as in the previous group, but with the exception that the two lower segment arteries instead of arising on either side of the aorta, have fused to form a common trunk, and have arisen from its anterior surface (*Fig.* 36).

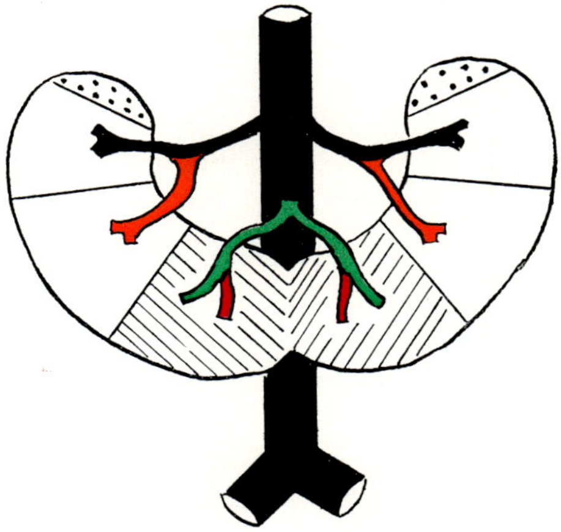

FIG. 36.—Type H-S IIb; the kidney substance tends to be fused across the midline and the lower segment arteries on both sides have fused, to take a common origin from the aorta.

Type H-S IIc

In those 'horse-shoe' kidneys where the solid substance of the kidney continues across the midline, in distinction to those whose lower poles are merely close in apposition, the posterior branch of the lower segment artery sometimes appears

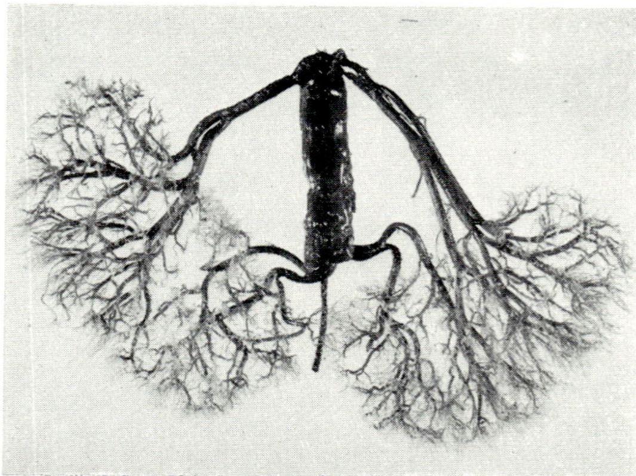

Fig. 37.—Type H-S IIc, a cast of a horse-shoe kidney of an adult. The apical, upper, middle, and posterior segment arteries are as in normal kidneys. The lower segment arteries on both sides not only arise from a common trunk from the aorta, but the posterior branches of the artery have arisen earlier, and outside the renal substance, and almost from the aorta direct.

outside the renal substance, and at first gives the impression of being a separate artery. Study, however, shows that it still retains its connexion with the anterior branch of the lower segment artery. The photograph of the cast in *Fig.* 37 illustrates this well. In these instances the posterior branch of the lower segment artery is often of a larger calibre, and it supplies a larger area than usual. In this, it does so at the expense of the posterior segment, which is correspondingly smaller.

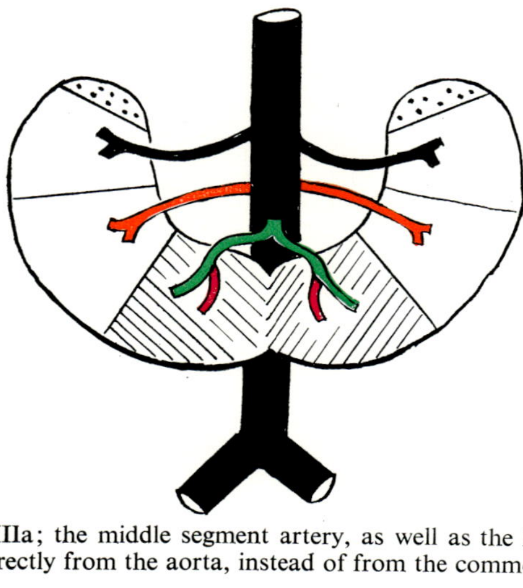

Fig. 38.—Type H-S IIIa; the middle segment artery, as well as the lower segment vessel, arises directly from the aorta, instead of from the common stem.

TYPE H-S IIIa

The arteries to the apical, upper, and posterior segments are as usual. The middle segment, however, tends to ape the lower segment artery in that it, too, has arisen direct from the aorta (*Fig.* 38).

TYPE H-S IIIb

A variation of the above type, particularly when there is a broad expanse of renal substance across the midline. Part of this latter and most dependent part of the

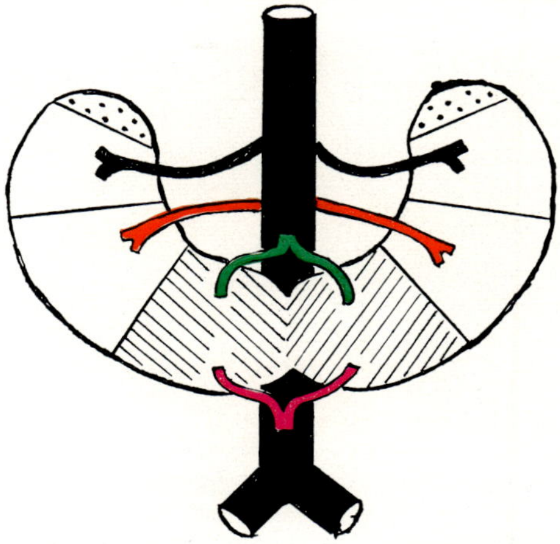

FIG. 39.—Type H-S IIIb, the lower poles of both kidneys are fused across the midline and receive twin vessels from the aorta both above and below the isthmus. The lower vessel, coloured in red, probably corresponds to the posterior branch of the lower segment artery.

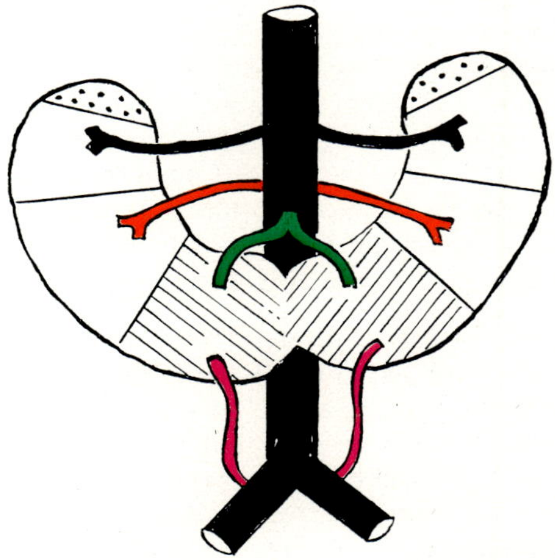

FIG. 40.—Type H-S IIIc, similar to the previous type, with the exception that the posterior branch of the lower segment artery (red) arises from the bifurcation of the aorta or the common iliac arteries.

kidney receives its blood-supply from a vessel which arises just above the isthmus, and part of it, that is the lower and posterior edge, is supplied by an artery which arises separately either from the aorta (*Fig.* 39), as a paired vessel from a single stem or as paired vessels from either side of the aorta. A third variation of the theme (Type H-S IIIc) is that these vessels supplying the dependent area of the 'horse-shoe' may arise, as shown in *Fig.* 40, from one or other iliac arteries. The question then arises as to whether these vessels are completely anomalous, or whether they are segmental vessels of the accepted pattern, but presenting in some new guise. Examination of the casts suggests the following explanation. In 'horse-shoe' kidneys such as these, the solid renal substance is wider but flattened since it is

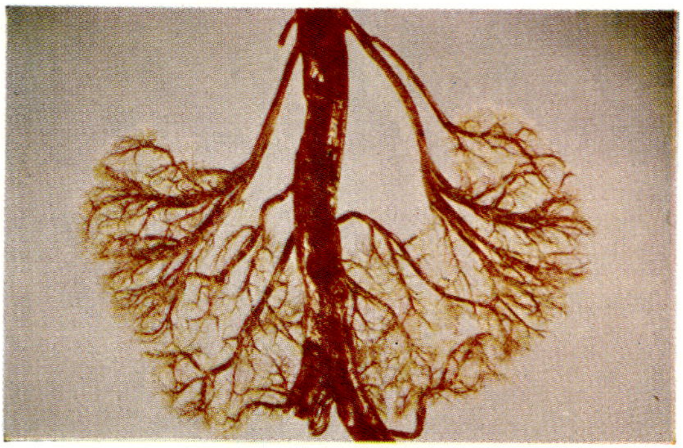

FIG. 41.—A colour photograph of a cast of an adult horse-shoe kidney, with considerable renal substance across the midline. It corresponds to Type H-S IIIc. The apical, upper, and posterior segment arteries are normal. The middle segments on both sides arise direct from the aorta. The anterior branches of the lower segment artery arise from a common trunk from the front of the aorta. The posterior branches of the lower segment on both sides arise from the right common iliac artery.

stretched over the aorta or its bifurcation. Indeed, the pelvi-calices of this area often have to drain 'up-and-over' the substance of the kidney. All this tends to push caudally, and rotate the area of tissue which would be normally the posterior part of the lower pole; that is, in other words, the area supplied by the posterior branch of the lower segment artery (*Fig.* 41). I suggest, therefore, that these vessels arising from the aorta or iliac arteries, below the isthmus of the kidney, are probably the posterior branches of the lower segment artery, which have taken their origin from the nearest point along the aortic route from which their mesonephric ancestors arose.

D. THE KIDNEY WHICH IS ABNORMAL IN SITE

Only one specimen was obtained in which the kidney lay within the bony pelvis, in the angle of the bifurcation of the aorta. It was smaller than normal, and was oval in shape. It appeared to have been quite functional (*Fig.* 42). It was supplied by three vessels of considerable calibre. One artery supplied the major part of the posterior surface; the other two were responsible for the anterolateral areas on either side. The posterior artery had a common origin with the right anterolateral artery, which arose from the bifurcation of the aorta. The left anterolateral artery arose from the left common iliac artery.

I have been unable, by study either of the casts or of the literature, to find any relation between the arterial structure of this kidney and those I have described previously.

COMMENT

It must be appreciated that from the relatively small series of casts studied, it has not been possible to cover every variation of the segmental arteries which one might encounter in anomalous renal states. I have been to some extent surprised

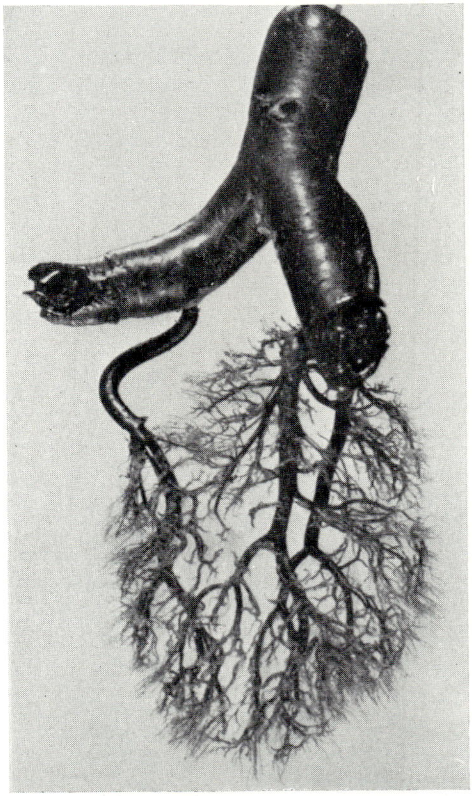

FIG. 42.—The posterior view of a cast of a pelvic kidney, lying in the angle of the bifurcation of the aorta. It is supplied by three arteries, two of which arose from the bifurcation of the aorta, the third arose from the left common iliac artery.

not only by the constancy of the arterial pattern, but also the finding that the variations tend to be ordered, and even predictable.

The purpose of this study has been partly to provide further anatomical knowledge, and partly to provide a guide which might be of assistance to the surgeon, in the operative field. It is true that an aortogram could be of considerable help as a preoperative measure to indicate the presence and course of the various arteries. In practice, however, such aortograms are often very difficult to interpret, and basic anatomical knowledge is a prerequisite. I have listed, therefore, the following comments, which are in no way dogmatic but which, in company with the previous descriptions, may be of some use to both surgeons and anatomists.

1. The upper, middle, and posterior segment arteries are the most constant in origin and position, and vary the least.

2. The lower segment artery is the most nomadic in its origin. If it arises directly from the aorta and originates cephalically (that is, near the main renal vessel), it will probably be small and supply its own segment only. If it arises more caudally, and near the origin of the genital vessel, it is likely to take the flow of both and give rise to the genital artery as well. Hence, a large lower segment artery may indicate that it supplies the gonad.

3. If the posterior branch of the lower segment artery originates separately from the anterior branch, it will most probably pass behind the ureter, the anterior branch passing in front.

4. In those instances where a vessel (which does not normally do so) takes an independent origin from the aorta, it may be larger in calibre and may effect a 'take-over' of part of the area of a neighbouring segment, which becomes correspondingly smaller.

5. When the renal substance extends in some solidarity over the aorta, the vessels which supply its combined lower poles may do so from both above and below the isthmus.

SUMMARY

1. The variations of the segmental arteries in the congenitally abnormal kidney tend to fall into an ordered pattern, and show a recognizable relationship to the five segments of the normal kidney.

2. Study of the embryology of the mesonephric arteries provides an explanation for these variations.

3. The nature of the segmental arteries, even in the extremes of variation, is the same as in the normal kidney—that is, there is no collateral circulation between the segments.

CHAPTER SIX

THE ANATOMY OF THE INTRARENAL ARTERIES IN DISEASE

THE previous studies have been confined to the study of the arterial anatomy in the normal and the congenitally abnormal kidney. The nature of the blood-supply and the discovery of the segmental arrangement of the intrarenal arteries has been described. In order, however, that this knowledge may be applied to the best advantage in the treatment of disease, it is necessary to study the effects of the disease upon the intrarenal vessels, and in particular to those lesions which tend to be localized and therefore amenable to surgical excision. A study was therefore made of the intrarenal vessels in kidneys affected by tumours, cysts, and calculous disease. Attempts were also made to study the effects of tuberculosis upon the vessels, but this proved to be virtually impossible, owing to the difficulty of obtaining post-mortem specimens in which the tuberculous lesion was sufficiently localized for the study to be of value. Likewise, operation specimens of tuberculous kidneys were too grossly affected by the disease to be of use.

THE SEGMENTAL ARTERIES IN TUMOURS AND CYSTS

The previous demonstration of the arterial pattern contributes to the knowledge and practice of surgery in two ways: first, by an addition to basic anatomical knowledge which is an essential for operative surgery, particularly a partial resection of the kidney; secondly, in its application to angiography in the diagnosis of disease.

Study of the vascular pattern in cysts and tumours has been done mainly because of the potential value of angiography in the differential diagnosis of these two conditions. Pyelography in such cases indicates that there is a mass compressing the calices which may be either cyst or tumour. At operation the nature of the lesion may be obvious, but sometimes inspection and palpation of the kidney yield little further information. Aortography is now becoming a more established procedure as a method of renal angiography, and many cases are reported in which the presence of a carcinoma of the renal parenchyma is indicated by 'pooling' of the radio-opaque dye which is believed to be lying in abnormal tumour vessels (Whiteside, 1953).

Other workers have shown that in contrast to neoplastic disease a solitary cyst indicates its presence by the absence of any dye in the area of the cyst which itself displaces the surrounding vessels. In a study of 500 cases in the literature, Walsh (1951), showed that in 7 per cent of apparently benign cysts, a malignant tumour was present in the cyst, and that where the contents of the cysts were haemorrhagic, the incidence of the associated neoplasm was as high as 30 per cent. Reagan and Carroll (1951) have described a case in which 'pooling' was seen around the

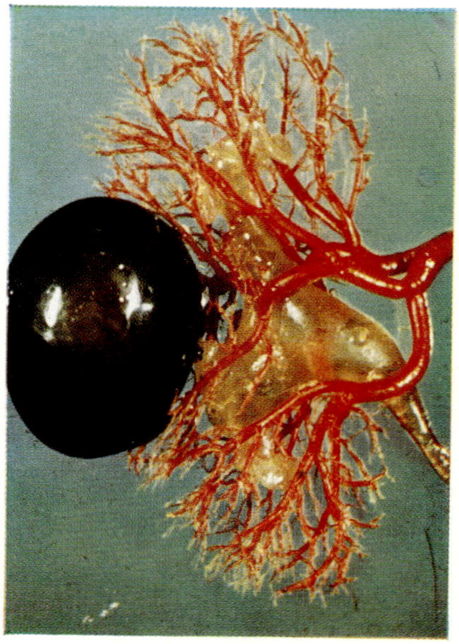

FIG. 43.—A cast of the right kidney seen from the front. The cyst in its lateral part has displaced downwards the middle segment artery, and displaced backwards the lateral branch of the artery to the upper segment. The pattern of the remaining segmental arteries is normal.

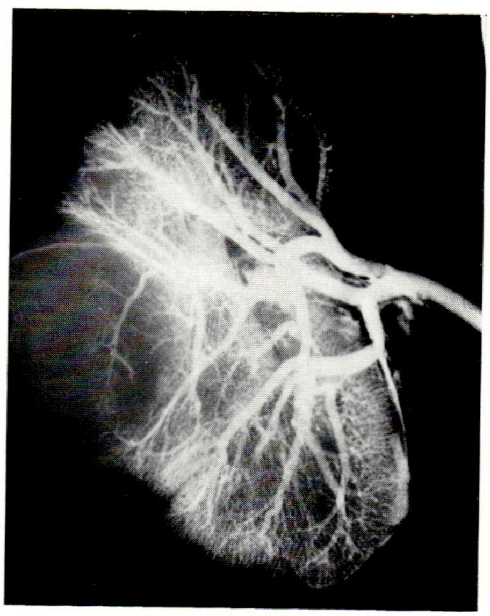

FIG. 44.—An arteriogram of the same kidney as seen in *Fig*. 43. All the segmental arteries can be seen. The cortical glomerular pattern extends to the very edge of the cyst. Contrast this with the arteriogram of a tumour in *Fig*. 50.

periphery of a cyst. Malignancy was therefore suspected and subsequently proved on histological examination.

Methods of Study

These were the same as in previous chapters. The angiography was done on operation and post-mortem specimens.

Cysts

A cast of a kidney with a solitary cyst on its lateral border is shown in *Fig*. 43. The cyst lies mainly in the middle and upper segments. The artery to the lower

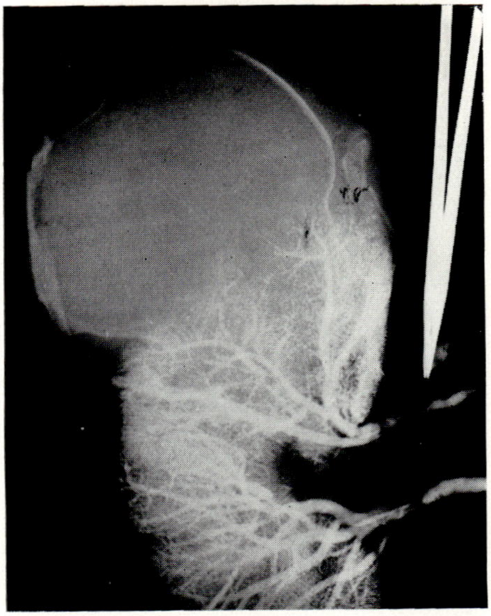

Fig. 45.—An arteriogram of a kidney with a large cyst at its upper pole. The arrangement of the segmental arteries is undisturbed, and the cortical pattern of the glomerular 'boutons' extends to the edge of the cyst. Contrast this also with *Fig*. 50.

segment arises as in Group I; the artery to the apical segment arises from the posterior division. The cyst has displaced downwards the middle segment artery and displaced backwards the lateral branch of the artery to the upper segment. Apart from this the arterial pattern is normal. The arteriogram (*Fig*. 44) confirms these facts, and, in addition, it shows that the normal cortical pattern with the glomerular 'boutons' extends right up to the edge of the cyst. With the exception of the avascular area occupied by the cyst itself, there is no diminution of the vascular supply.

Fig. 45 shows an arteriogram of a kidney which had a large cyst at its upper pole. All the segmental vessels are intact, but the upper branches of the arteries to the apical, upper, and posterior segments are to some extent flattened by the cyst. Again, a normal cortical pattern with well-marked 'boutons' extends to the edge of the cyst which itself is avascular.

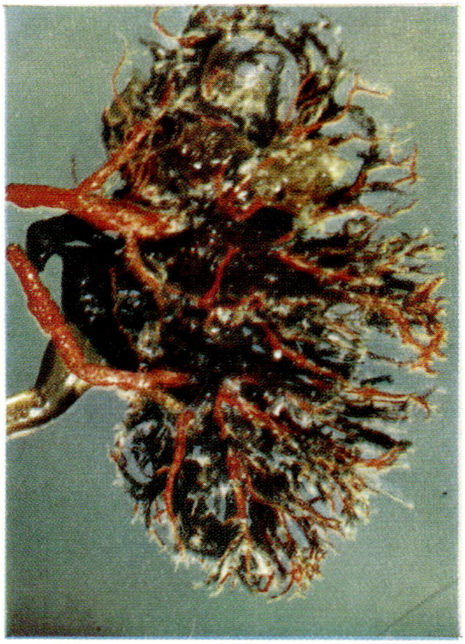

FIG. 46.—A cast of the left kidney seen from the front. There was a small carcinoma at the upper pole. In this area the vascular supply is diminished and the apical branch of the artery to the upper segment is absent, due to destruction by the tumour.

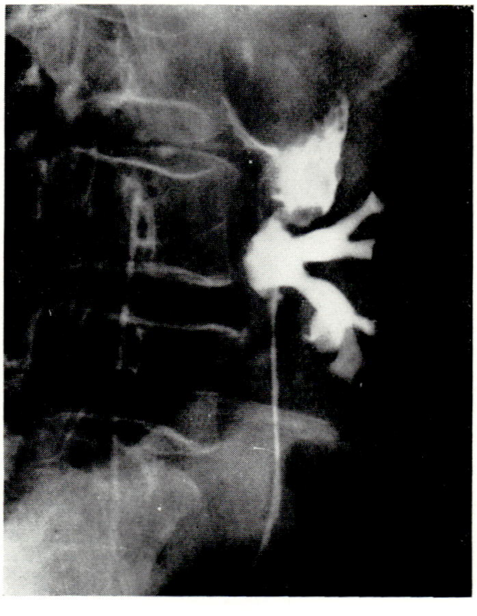

FIG. 47.—An ascending pyelogram of the same kidney as seen in *Fig.* 46.

Carcinoma of the Kidney (Hypernephroma)

Three specimens illustrate tumours of early, middle, and advanced degrees of growth.

The Early Growth

Fig. 46 shows a cast of a kidney in which there was a carcinoma at the upper pole. The growth was small and at operation the kidney looked normal, but a mass could be felt at its upper pole. The presence of the tumour had been diagnosed on the history of haematuria and a deformity of the upper calyx on pyelography (*Fig.* 47). The cast shows the site of the tumour in the upper and apical segments,

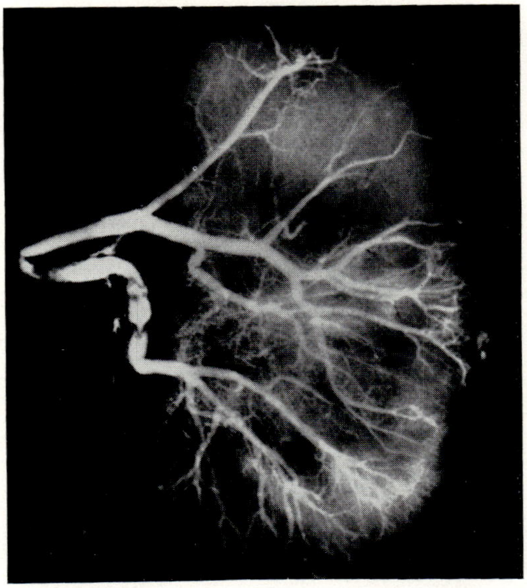

Fig. 48.—An arteriogram of the same kidney shown in *Figs.* 46 and 47. It shows the area in the upper pole where the blood-supply is diminished, the apical branch of the upper segment being absent due to destruction by the growth. There is no cortical glomerular filling in the region of the tumour. Contrast this with the cysts in *Figs.* 44 and 45.

the calix being compressed by the growth. The veins in the area are intact and their normal pattern is little disturbed. The arterial supply to the area, however, is diminished, and the smaller branches of the segmental vessels are arranged around the tumour like 'grasping fingers'. The arteriogram confirms the findings of the cast (*Fig.* 48), showing that the apical branch of the artery to the upper segment is absent, the lateral branch being intact. The glomerular pattern in the neighbourhood of the tumour is absent.

The Growth of Middle Degree

Fig. 49 is a photograph of a specimen with a carcinoma at its lower pole. The growth is of moderate size and its cut surface has a characteristic appearance.

The arteriogram (*Fig*. 50) shows a normal distribution and pattern of the segmental vessels in the upper half of the kidney, for the arteries to the apical and upper

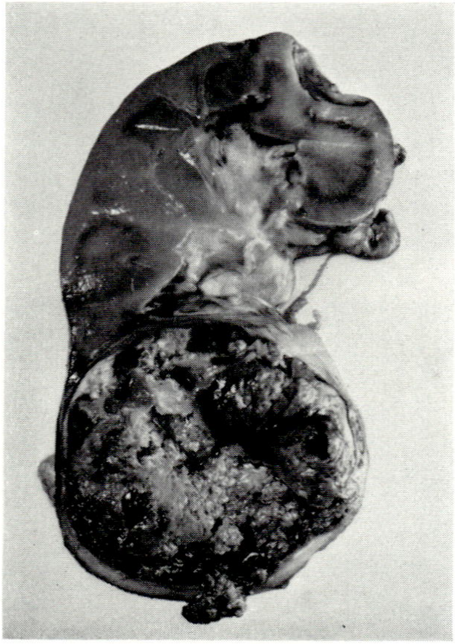

FIG. 49.—A specimen of a kidney with a carcinoma at its lower pole.

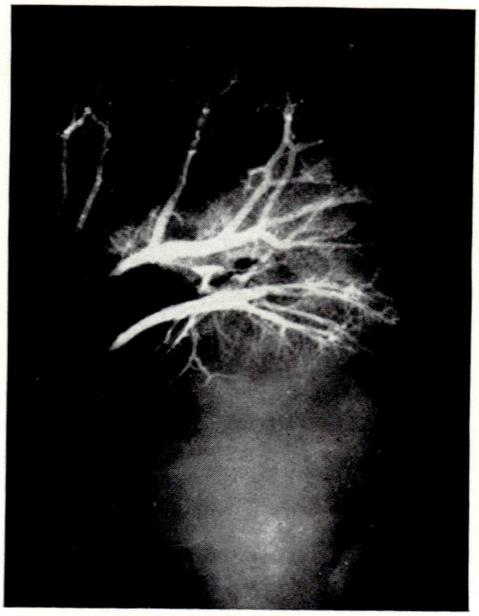

FIG. 50.—The arteriogram of the same kidney seen in *Fig*. 49. The segmental pattern of the arteries is normal in the upper half of the kidney. In the area occupied by the tumour there are no segmental vessels present. Note how the branches of the arteries nearest the tumour are spread over its dome.

segments, and also the upper branches of the posterior segment, are well defined. The artery to the posterior segment is present, but its branches are displaced so as to follow the convex curve of the tumour. The remaining segmental vessels have disappeared, and the site occupied by the tumour itself is avascular. In the area which forms the junction of normal kidney tissue with that of the tumour the branches of the neighbouring segmental vessels are pushed apart so that they appear to hold the tumour like 'grasping fingers'. In contrast to the benign cyst, however, *the cortical glomerular pattern is not evident in this transitional zone between tumour and normal kidney.*

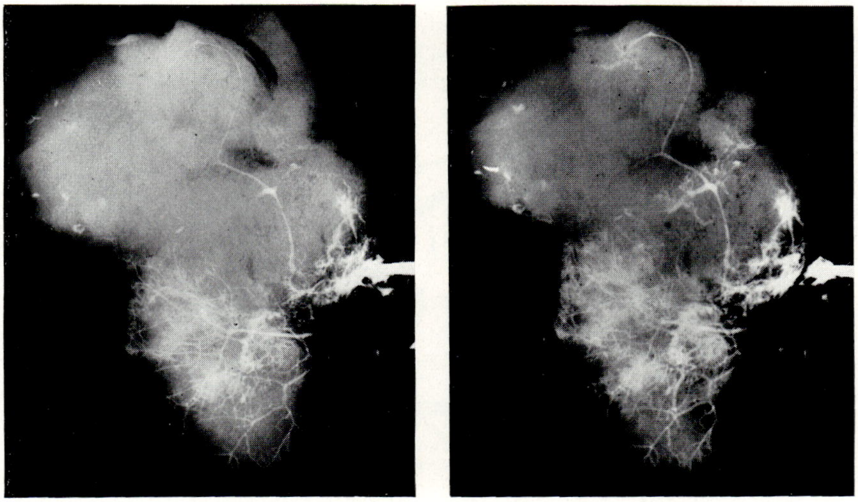

A B

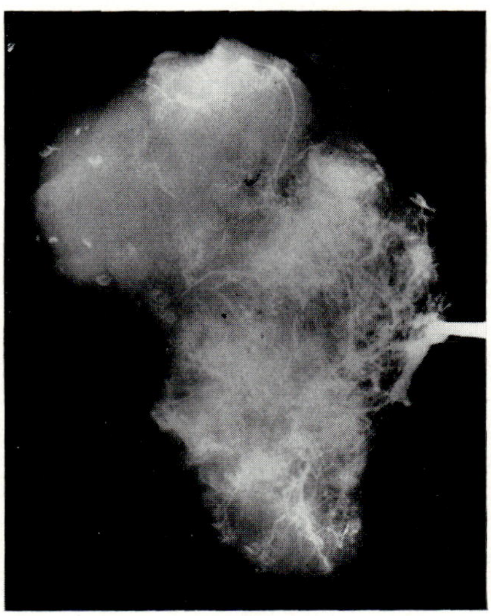

C

FIG. 51.—An arteriogram of an advanced case of carcinoma of the kidney. The bulk of the tumour was at the upper pole, where there is no arterial filling. No 'pooling' is seen in the arterial phase of the injection (A), but it can be seen slightly in the early venous phase (B), and to a greater extent in the later venous phase of the last film (C).

The Advanced Growth

Fig. 51A is an arteriogram of a large carcinoma of the kidney, in which growth was visible in the mouth of the main renal vein. The calibre of the intrarenal arteries is small and the normal segmental pattern is not discernible. This lack of recognizable pattern was thought to be due to the presence of nodules of growth in various parts of the kidney, and subsequent histological examination proved this to be so. The bulk of the growth lies at the upper pole, where there is little or no arterial filling. Two more films, taken some five and ten seconds later (*Fig.* 51B, C), by which time the dye is leaving the arterial side and entering the venous phase, show evidence of 'pooling', especially in the mid-zone of the organ.

These pictures show some of the arteriographic appearances of renal cysts and tumours. The area occupied by the cyst is avascular, but the segmental arterial pattern is undisturbed and the cortical pattern is normal and extends to the very edge of the cyst.

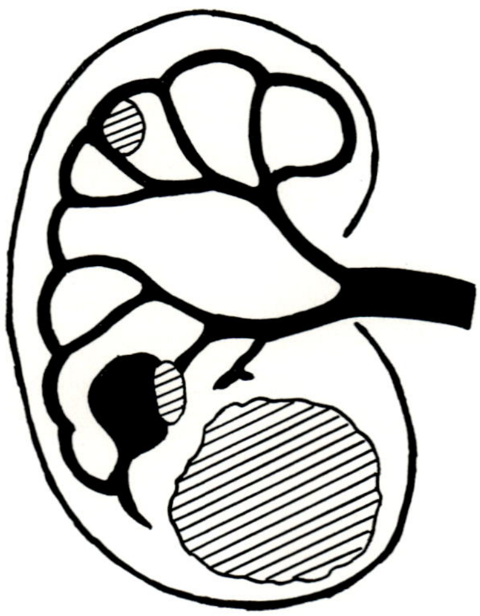

FIG. 52.—A diagram which illustrates my theory of the mechanism of the 'pooling' of opaque dye, which is sometimes seen in arteriograms of carcinoma of the kidney. When the tumour invades the veins, secondary growths obstruct the venous arcades and produce local dilatation of these thin-walled vessels, due to back-pressure. The drainage of the dye from these areas is slower—hence the 'pooling'.

The appearances of the carcinoma have not been uniform, but to some extent this may be due to the difference in the degree of growth. In all three specimens the area occupied by the tumour is avascular, with corresponding distortion or absence of the segmental vessels. In the two earlier growths the arteries in the zone between tumour and normal kidney have been distorted by the tumour to appear like 'grasping fingers' but, unlike the cysts, the cortical pattern is absent in the immediate vicinity of the tumour.

The presence of 'pooling' was noticed only in the specimen of advanced growth, in whose preoperative translumbar aortogram it was also noted. It should be recalled, however, that the 'pooling' was not seen in the arterial phase of the experimental angiography, but only in the later venous phases.

Comment

It is well known that hypernephroma invades the renal veins, a fact which is not surprising when one examines the extensive venous system of arcades, as shown by the casts in *Figs*. 21 and 22 (pp. 25, 26). It has already been shown that the venous system within the kidney has a free anastomosis. Now, I suggest that this venous pathway within the substance of the kidney provides not only the method of spread for external metastases, but also a method of spread within the kidney itself, for such a free anastomosis provides an 'open back-door' to every segment in the organ. *Fig*. 52 is a diagram indicating my theory that the 'pooling' so often noted in angiograms of renal tumours is produced not by the collection of the dye in abnormal vessels in the tumour, but by delayed emptying in the intrarenal venous system, which results from partial obstruction of the veins, caused by nodules of growth within their lumen. If my theory proves to be correct, then the presence of 'pooling' may be a guide to prognosis.

CALCULOUS DISEASE

In planning the site of resection of the kidney substance for calculous disease, two factors must be considered. The extent of the calicine disease and the arterial segments which are involved.

The stone, and also the diseased calicine bed in which it has matured, must be removed, for as Hamilton Stewart (1952) points out, if the deformed 'nest' or 'sump' in which the stone has matured is not included in the resected portion, it will be a nesting ground for future stone formation and, if infected, will maintain infection in the urinary tract.

The second factor, concerning the arterial segments, presents a further problem, for although the distribution, pattern, and nature of the blood-supply in the healthy kidney have been investigated, it is not known whether they will remain unaltered in a kidney affected by calculous disease. Since partial nephrectomy is being proposed for treatment of this, it is of importance to know to what extent the segmental arteries may be altered in the diseased kidney.

An investigation was therefore carried out to answer the following questions:—

1. Is the arrangement of the segmental arteries disturbed in calculous disease?
2. Is there any alteration in the calibre of the main segmental arteries?
3. Is there any alteration in the finer vessels in the cortex, particularly in those areas where the calculus lies or has been formed?

Material for Investigation

Both operation and post-mortem specimens were used. In order to satisfy the criteria necessary for adequate investigation, the kidney specimen had to be intact, with the stone in position and sufficient length of renal artery present to ensure that all segmental arteries, however precocious their origin, would be included. This last requirement gave rise to difficulty with regard to operation specimens, since it was not always possible for surgeons to remove the kidney with enough pedicle to include all the origins of the segmental arteries from the main stem. It was necessary, therefore, in some cases to cannulate a divided vessel separately if it had been accidentally separated from the main stem during the process of nephrectomy. The post-mortem specimens, however, always included part of the aorta.

It was decided to include all degrees of calculous disease in the investigation. A kidney with a small stone would be the most interesting as regards any change in the fine cortical vessels near the lesion, but such a specimen would be difficult to obtain. A calculous hydronephrosis on the other hand would have less interest as to the fine cortical vessels, but would be of more value as to alteration of pattern and calibre of the segmental arteries. Eleven cases are included in this series.

The specimens were collected from a number of hospitals and post-mortem rooms in the London area.

Methods of Investigation

The same methods and technique were used as in the earlier experiments. Renal arteriograms were made first, and later a plastic cast was made of the arterial and calicine systems. In the latter case, the calculus became embedded in the resin, except where it was adherent to the wall of the calix, or lay in a space which had no communication with the pelvi-calicine system.

Technique of Corrosion

Corrosion had been carried out satisfactorily with specimens of normal kidneys by immersion of the specimen in concentrated hydrochloric acid. The same technique, when carried out with specimens containing stone, resulted in solution of the calculus where this was not entirely surrounded and protected by the resin. Innumerable experiments were made, using various fluids, in order to find a satisfactory corrosive agent which would remove the organic tissue, but leave intact the calculus and the resin. Dilute acid and 20 per cent cold caustic soda were unsatisfactory, as were attempts at removal of the organic matrix by digestion, using suitably buffered solutions of trypsin, pepsin, papain, and also bacterial decomposition. Finally a satisfactory result was obtained by boiling the specimen in 4*N* caustic soda. The manufacturers of the resin had expressed doubt as to whether the resin would be able to resist caustic soda at this temperature, but after a preliminary trial with a block of resin, it was found that satisfactory removal of the organic material was obtained, without damage to either the resin cast or the calculi.

Composition and Formation of Calculus

Examination of the specimens has produced some evidence as to the mode of formation of renal calculus.

Most staghorn calculi lying in the pelvis of the kidney suggest by their shape that they have resulted from growth of a small stone which was initially unable to enter the ureter because of its shape or size. Such a calculus, in the course of time, shows projections upon its surface at points opposite the mouths of the major calices, indicating that urinary deposition is laid down in the line of the current of urine in the same way as silt forms on the islets of a delta at the mouth of a large river.

A single stone, occupying and taking the shape of a calix (*Fig.* 53), because of its conical shape, will never pass into the pelvis. The cast of the remaining calices show these to be normal. Such a case would be suitable for partial nephrectomy, removing the diseased stone and calix at the junction of the latter with its normal fellows. This stone, as do many others, shows the close adhesion of the stone to the wall of the calix. Such evidence as there is suggests that this adhesion is secondary, and not the primary attachment of the stone to the pyramid, as Randall (1937) described. It is more probable that a smaller calculus or concretion was extruded into the lumen of the calix but being too large to pass the isthmus leading to the

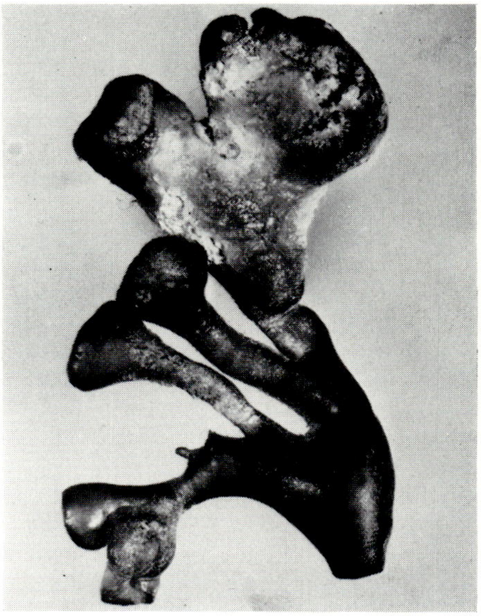

FIG. 53.—A cast of the pelvi-calicine system of the right kidney. The upper major calix contains and is almost completely filled by a stone which is embedded in the resin. The remainder of the calices are normal.

major calix, remained in its parent cavity where urinary salts were deposited upon it from above downwards, as with a stalagmite, until it has assumed the shape of the calix and to some extent that of the pyramid itself.

Although many staghorn calculi are so gross as to provide little information, most of those examined in this series have yielded some evidence of value.

A specimen, with a gross staghorn calculus of considerable density, filled the pelvis and all the calices of the kidney. Radiography, however, showed that opacities were present in the lower and middle segments which lay outside the calicine system. These opacities differed entirely from the smooth continuous density of the calculus within the calicine system, in that they were composed of innumerable fine granules.

Another specimen illustrated an earlier phase in the development of calculus (*Fig.* 54A). A large stone was present in part of the pelvis and in the lower major calix. In its substance were seen a number of concretions which were oval in shape. In the region of the pyramids there were no less than 18 similar oval opacities lying in two main groups, the larger in the middle segment, the smaller in the lower segment. In contrast most of the opacities embedded in the central calculus were

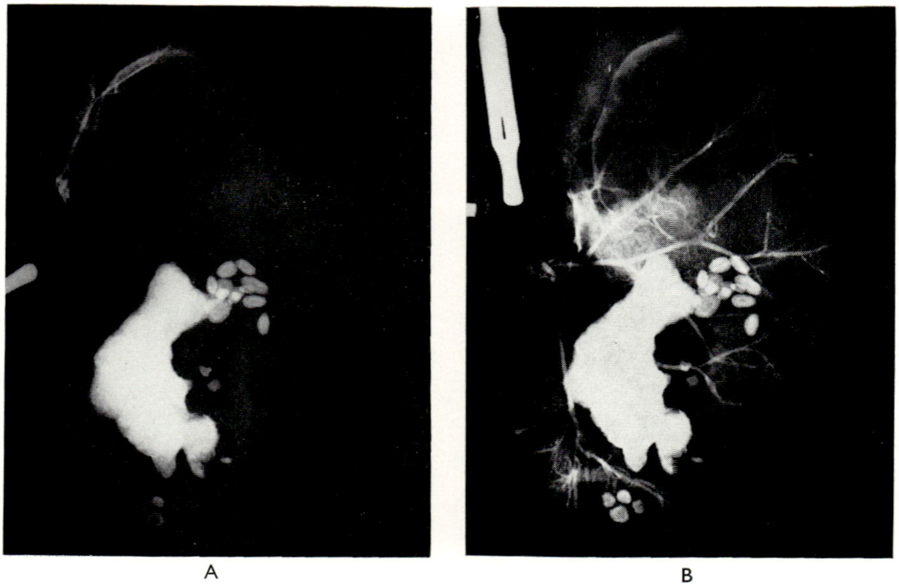

FIG. 54.—A, The radiograph of a kidney with a staghorn calculus. There are a number of oval laminated stones in the middle and lower segments. An arteriogram has been made of the apical segment. B, The arteriogram of all the segments except the apical segment. Note the oval opacities which can be seen embedded in the lower part of the staghorn calculus.

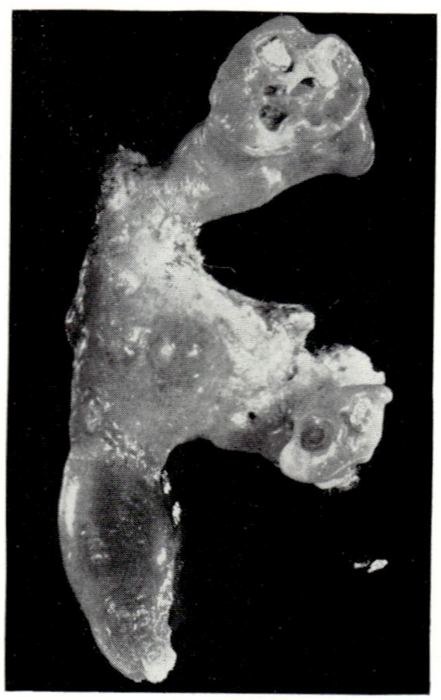

FIG. 55.—A cast of the pelvi-calicine system of the same kidney as seen in *Fig.* 54. Note the laminated oval opacity embedded in the middle calix, and also the depressions in the cast caused by other oval calculi.

in its lowest part. This, I think, was probably produced by gravity, for although the concretions had most likely arisen from the more prolific middle segment, they had fallen to the dependent calix and become embedded there. Even though these concretions were small, they were laminated in structure, their size varying from 3 to 6 mm. in their longest axis. Comparison of the cast and the radiograph, however, showed that some of these oval opacities were probably in the cortex, since only a few were embedded in the side wall of the calicine cast (*Fig.* 55), the remainder having fallen free in the process of corrosion, being unprotected by the resin in the calix.

Laminations even in so small a concretion as 4 mm. lying outside the calicine system suggest that successive deposition of salts can occur without the contact of urine.

A third specimen contained a large calculus, the bulk of which was homogeneous, but opposite the major calices were ring shadows similar to those described in the previous specimen. Their position suggested that concretions or further stones had been produced after the formation of the main calculus and, having been extruded from its parent calix, it became embedded in the growing pelvic stone. That such calculi are constantly being formed is shown by the presence of innumerable small stones in the periphery of the kidney substance, some being within the calicine system and others outside it, in the cortex of the kidney.

These are seen both in the radiograph and on examination of the cast to be quite separate from the main calculus.

Comment

The pathogenesis of renal calculus, particularly that of the early lesion, is still obscure. In 1937 Randall made a microscopical examination of a number of kidneys and observed that in 28 cases small stones were adherent to, or growing upon the renal papillae. He made serial histological sections of papillae and described the 'initiating lesion' or 'milk patch', associated with his name. The patch consisted of a deposit of calcium in an area which became progressively more fibrotic and avascular, but which lacked any microscopical evidence of inflammation.

Randall's theory has now been challenged by Carr (1954), who has shown that in normal kidneys minute concretions of varying size can be found in the parenchyma in the region of the fornices of the calices and also in the corticomedullary zone, and immediately under the capsule of the kidney. These concretions may be multiple and are increased in number and size in calculous disease. Radiological examination of a calculus removed by myself, at partial nephrectomy, showed it to consist of similar minute concretions.

Carr suggests that these concretions form in the lymphatics of the kidney, the normal flow of lymph being from the periphery towards the hilum. He postulates that renal calculi form as the result of obstruction of the lymphatics in the region of the caliceal fornices, the concretions being held up at this point from which they subsequently erupt into the caliceal lumen.

As little is known as yet about the lymphatics of the kidney, part of Carr's explanation is necessarily theoretical. It is, however, strongly supported by his observation that the minute concretions are sometimes seen to lie in a chain, the smaller ones being near the periphery of the organ.

Although my own work has been concerned primarily with the study of the intrarenal arteries, it was impossible to do this without taking some interest in the disease process affecting the kidney which was under study. I have recorded my observations, for some of them do have some bearing upon the aetiology of calculus. Calculi have been found in the parenchyma of the kidney, lying outside the lumen of the calices. The arrangement, size, shape, and number of these opacities varied. In some they consisted of innumerable fine granules, packed

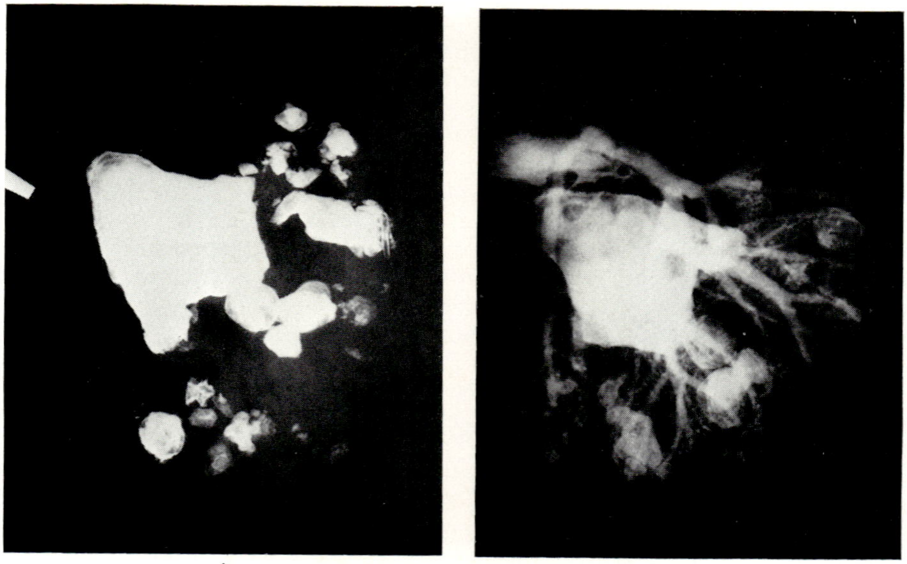

A B

FIG. 56.—A, The radiograph of a kidney with a large stone in the pelvis. There are a number of smaller stones in the major and minor calices. The majority of the smaller stones lie nearer the periphery of the kidney. Note the pencillated and laminated opacity near the periphery of the middle segment. B, The arteriogram of the same kidney. There is no diminution in the size of the segmental arteries.

closely together and being of approximately equal size; in others the collections were more loosely associated, the individual granules varying in size and shape and often being some distance from one another, the largest bodies lying near the calices, the smallest nearer the periphery.

Some of these opacities were oval in shape, being of remarkable similarity even in different specimens. This shape and that of the pencillated body illustrated in *Fig*. 56, suggest, as does Carr, that these minute calculi are formed in some tube or duct within the kidney substance, possibly in the lymphatic system. Although in one specimen the opacities were confined to two segments only, in many specimens they were distributed evenly throughout the substance of the kidney.

Recurrence of the calculus is not only due to inadequate removal of the stone at the initial operation, but also due to the continued formation of further calculi. This has been demonstrated not only by the combined presence of the staghorn calculus in the pelvis of the kidney and smaller stones in the parenchyma, but also by the staghorn itself containing in its substance those small oval calculi which have been extruded from time to time from the parenchyma into the calices.

Similar evidence is shown in a specimen of a kidney, in my series, from which a calculus had been removed some years previously. The subsequent examination of the kidney and cast showed that it contained four groups of composite stones, in two of which the smaller granules lay near the periphery of the kidney. Again, the central stone in the pelvis contained many smaller calculi. This provided yet

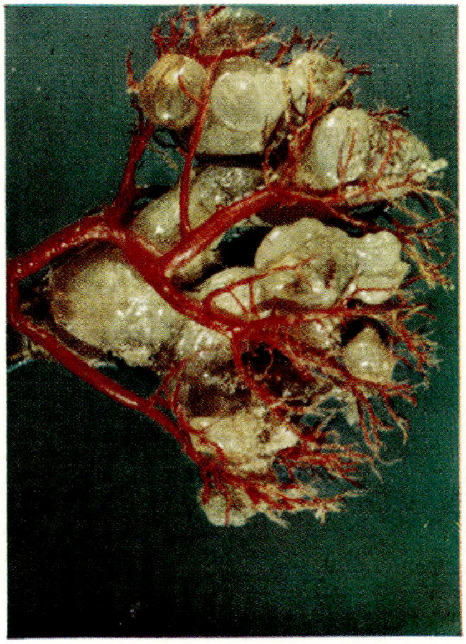

FIG. 57.—The anterior view of the cast of the same kidney as seen in *Fig.* 56. There are a number of calculi embedded in the resin. Note the normal segmental pattern of the arteries; their calibre is within normal limits.

further evidence that tiny stones or 'concretions'—call them what you will—start in the periphery of the kidney, and gradually migrate through the cortical substance towards the collecting calices, into which they erupt. Once there, they may, if the calix is normal and the pelvi-ureteric junction is large enough, be washed out with the ebb and flow of urinary peristalsis. If not, then they may grow as does the stalactite, due to deposition of salts, or become embedded in a larger calculus which is already in the calix, like a fossil caught in mesozoic mud.

In my series of specimens one observation was made, which is not recorded by Carr. Some of the small opacities, particularly the oval bodies, show lamination. As some of these bodies are found in the cortex, and not in the calyces, how then do they obtain their laminations? If you believe that the most likely cause of lamination is successive deposition of urinary salts, then since the tiny 'stone' is in the cortex and not in official contact with urine, one has little option but to feel, as I do, that these tiny stones probably start their existence in the renal tubules. If you find this theory unreasonable, then the only alternative is to say that the lymph of the kidney is subject to considerable electrolyte variation—but this would involve an equally considerable study of the renal lymph!

The Segmental Arteries in Calculous Disease

Segmental Pattern

There was remarkably little disturbance in the distribution and arrangement of the intrarenal arteries, the pattern being little changed from that as described in the normal kidney. Even when hydronephrosis was present, the calices being grossly dilated and containing calculi, the segmental arteries were not displaced, and indeed the caliceal dilatations appeared to have grown around them (*Fig.* 57).

Calibre of the Segmental Arteries

In one case (*see Fig.* 54B) the calibre of the segmental arteries was reduced to approximately half the normal size. This case was an operation specimen and as the renal arteriogram was made within an hour of removal, it was thought that this reduction in the calibre might be due to spasm of the vessels possessing residual life. Subsequent specimens were therefore not investigated until at least twenty-four hours after operation, it being thought that by this time all cellular activity would have ceased and the investigation results would be comparable with those done on normal kidneys.

Apart from this one specimen, the investigation showed little change in the calibre of the segmental vessels and their main branches (*see Fig.* 56B). In calculous hydronephrosis the vessels were normal or slightly reduced in size.

The Arterial Pattern in the Cortex

The pattern of the finer cortical vessels in the segments of the kidney showed considerable change compared with the normal. The cortical vessels, although still discernible, were frail and lacked the contrast and definition seen in the films of normal kidneys (*see Figs.* 18, 54B). This lack of solidarity was often most evident in the region where the stone was present, the finer vessels being elongated and tortuous, especially when the cortex was particularly avascular. It was also noticeable that the normal 'boutons' could not be seen.

CHAPTER SEVEN

THE ANATOMY OF OPERATIVE TECHNIQUE

SURGERY of the kidney was confined for many years to lithotomy and nephrectomy. This, of course, was due partly to the prevalence of stone, partly to the fact that the kidney is a bilateral organ only one of which is necessary for life, and partly to the dictates of early anaesthesia which necessitated that operations must be both quick and simple.

The advance of modern anaesthesia, our increased knowledge of pathology and biochemistry, and, not least, the advent of chemotherapy, have given surgeons the opportunity to reconsider time-honoured procedures and to seek for methods which, though less conservative in principle, will aim at greater conservation of normal tissue.

In the main, advances and interest have been centred upon three aspects of renal surgery—partial nephrectomy, hydronephrosis, and the surgical aspects of renal hypertension. Increased knowledge of the details of the renal anatomy and circulation, the physiology of the action of the renal pelvis, and experimental and clinical work on hypertension, have aided this activity.

PARTIAL NEPHRECTOMY

That removal of one kidney is a satisfactory treatment for localized disease provided that its fellow can carry out the work of both, is a traditional action, but *it makes no provision for the possibility that many of the diseases which affect the kidney are potentially bilateral.* Removal of one kidney including much normal tissue for the sake of excision of a localized area of disease is therefore an unsatisfactory policy in that it removes much 'reserve of normal tissue' which in future years may ill be spared. In those cases in which nephrectomy has been done, partial nephrectomy becomes an operation of necessity when disease presents itself again in the remaining kidney. How much better it would have been, therefore, to have removed only diseased tissue, instead of the whole kidney, in the first instance.

Partial nephrectomy therefore is a logical operation. It is essential, however, to remember that although partial nephrectomy may be the operation of preference in the treatment of localized disease, it should also be one of selection, for not every case is necessarily suitable. As Riches (1960) has emphasized, partial nephrectomy can be an appropriate operation for *some* examples of the following renal conditions: stone, caliceal diverticulum, cyst, hydronephrosis, tuberculosis, injury, tumour, and localized infection. To this list I personally would add the occasional case of renal hypertension, where this is due to scarring from previous disease or injury.

In making the decision as to the type of surgical treatment, it is therefore necessary to consider the disease both from the viewpoint of the pathology and the operation. The criteria which must be satisfied in the production of sound treatment are:—

1. A low mortality.
2. A low morbidity.
3. Freedom from recurrence of the disease.

The first two of these criteria are very largely the concern of a satisfactory operative surgical technique, with the aim of preventing, if possible, two of the chief complications—postoperative haemorrhage and urinary leak from the cut surface of the kidney. Both these troubles can be acute in the immediate postoperative period, and can contribute to mortality; likewise they can be persistent, with chronic urinary flow from the wound and a perpetual bleeding either from the raw surface of the incision into the kidney tissue, or by haematuria through the normal urinary outflow.

The third factor—that of prevention of recurrence of disease—is a more complex matter.

Freedom from Recurrence of Disease

At first sight this can be easily satisfied by partial nephrectomy; a little thought, and especially practical experience, teaches that the whole matter, like many others in nature, life, and surgery, is largely a compromise. The surgical approach must embrace:—

1. A sufficiently radical removal of tissue to include the disease and a margin of normal tissue.
2. Conservation of every available piece of normal functional kidney tissue that remains.
3. Avoidance of nephrectomy by every possible means.
4. A surgical technique combining maximum haemostasis, and avoidance of leaving ischaemic tissue in the remaining portion of the kidney.

These basic principles, however, will be influenced by the individual diseases, and even then, since it is impossible to legislate for every presentation of a problem, the treatment of individual cases will have to be settled on their own merits. Despite this, perhaps, the following notes on the various presentations of disease, may be of some practical use.

STONE

If you accept that the evidence presented in the previous chapters is valid, then the treatment must involve:—

1. Removal of the stone, complete.
2. Excision of the 'stone nest'—that is, the diseased calix in which the stone has grown, as advocated by Hamilton Stewart, for this, with its fibrotic and often granulomatous wall, will only hatch out another stone, or at best be a source of chronic infection in the urinary tract.
3. Removal of the adjacent cortex, if there is evidence on radiograph or past history, or even perhaps suspicion, that behind the base of the stone there are further concretions (though diminishing progressively in size) steadily migrating towards the calix.

With these principles in mind, the treatment of stone will also depend upon the presentation of the problem, which can be in the following ways:—

1. Simple Stone in the Pelvis of the Kidney

Providing there is no other evidence of stone in the kidney, that the calices are normal, that there is no previous history of disease, and no indication from which segment the stone may have arisen, a simple removal of the stone from the pelvis is quite justified.

2. Stone in the Calix

If this is in the upper or lower poles, removal of the affected calix, with its stone and the surrounding area of cortex, in general will suffice.

3. Stone in the Calix, with Evidence of Concretions in the Cortex

As with the previous case, a partial nephrectomy should be done—removing stone, calix, and diseased cortex. There is a problem which sometimes arises. A stone is found in the lower calix, but the radiograph suggests that the stone has probably arisen from the upper calix. It is reasonable to assume that it is the upper segment which is at fault, and that the stone has fallen by gravity into the lower calix. This being so, it is probably better to remove the diseased upper segment by partial nephrectomy, and at the same time remove the stone from the lower calix through the upper pole of the kidney. If, as sometimes happens, but less often, I think, the middle segment is diseased, then a rather more extensive 'lower pole partial nephrectomy' will usually cope with the problem.

4. Small Staghorn Calculus

For this, removal of either upper or lower pole of the kidney is advised, depending on the size of the stone and its predominance in either pole. The choice of the segment of kidney to be removed may also be influenced, not only by the stone itself, but also by whether there is any *evidence as to where the stone may first have formed.* Small stones, or concretions, as in *Fig.* 54B, in a segment, strongly indicate the route of approach to the staghorn and the area of cortex to be removed.

5. Large Staghorn Calculus and Bilateral Staghorn Calculi

In these cases it is evident that the disease process has passed beyond the possibility of radical cure; therefore I think the object of treatment should be removal of the staghorn, with the minimum amount of damage to the kidney, and at the same time leaving the maximum amount of functioning kidney tissue in the body. From practical experience in the operating theatre and from study of the vascular supply of the kidney in the laboratory, I have no great faith in the 'bloodless field' along Brodel's line. It is the veins—those longitudinal systems, row upon row (*see Fig.* 22, p. 26) of venous arcades—which give the trouble, not so much the arteries. I think that 'splitting' the kidney is fraught with danger. I have devised a method, which so far has always been successful, of removing even the largest staghorn calculus by partial nephrectomy. This is described in a later paragraph on surgical technique.

TUBERCULOSIS

Renal tuberculosis is, of course, part of a generalized disease so the treatment of it must be both general and local. The selective combined medical-surgical treatment of urogenital tuberculosis was introduced as a parallel to the treatment of pulmonary tuberculosis (Semb, 1949). Medical treatment aims at the therapy of the non-destructive infiltrations of the urogenital tract, whereas surgery is utilized for removal of necrotic or destructive foci of the ulcerocavernous type. In the last ten years I have followed the principles laid down by Semb (1955):—

1. Parenchymatous lesions: medical treatment.
2. Local destructive lesions (where foci are limited to approximately two-thirds of the kidney): partial nephrectomy after previous general treatment including chemotherapy.
3. Advanced renal tuberculosis: nephrectomy.

As with pulmonary lesions, the presence of non-destructive tuberculosis in the remaining part of the kidney and superficial change in the pelvis, ureter, and bladder are not contra-indications to operation, as these will often heal secondarily, or as the result of chemotherapy. Of Semb's 251 cases of renal tuberculosis, partial nephrectomy was done in 128 cases (51 per cent—141 resections). Bilateral partial nephrectomy was done in 13 out of 16 cases of bilateral disease with local destructive lesions. Eighty-nine per cent of these patients subsequently had tubercle-free urine. Semb had few complications and no postoperative deaths.

PRINCIPLES OF OPERATIVE TECHNIQUE

Pyelolithotomy

Many textbooks of surgery advocate that when removing a stone from the pelvis of the kidney, the latter should be incised on its posterior surface, and that the incision should be across the pelvis—that is, by a slightly curved incision, approximately parallel to the hilum. Others suggest an incision at right-angles to the hilum. In theory, the posterior part of the pelvis is the most suitable place for incision, since it is least likely to be obscured by arteries. I must emphasize, however, that care must be taken not to extend the incision in the pelvis too far into the hilum, for under its lip, although often quite easily visible, lies the posterior division of the renal artery, as it sweeps across the pelvis to terminate in the posterior segment artery (*Figs*. 5B, 8B, 13B, pp. 9, 10, 15).

In practice, I believe in incising the pelvis wherever it is most easily accessible, be it on its anterior or posterior surface, or even through its inferior margin. In many cases the anterior segment arteries do not arise from the main renal artery until the latter reaches the hilum, and it is perfectly safe to incise the pelvis on its anterior surface, providing care is taken to avoid the segmental arteries. The posterior approach to the pelvis always involves mobilization of the kidney, a procedure which, however gentle, is not without its effect on the blood-pressure and on the biochemical disturbance of the renal function; whereas, if the anterior approach is feasible, and gives adequate access, in the individual patient, the latter is spared the trauma of mobilization of the organ.

Partial Nephrectomy

The previous work has shown that the distribution of the arteries within the kidney forms a pattern which is constant, and upon this is founded the division of the renal parenchyma into five segments.

There is no collateral arterial supply between these segments. Ligation of a segmental artery will affect only that segment and it will not produce ischaemia nor interference with the blood-supply of the neighbouring segments. This lack of arterial anastomosis will render the technique of resection easier since the field of operation will be relatively bloodless, following the ligation of the segmental artery. This is borne out by Eberhart and Banks (1952) who found that ligation of the artery supplying the area of operation produced an almost bloodless field.

Lastly, it should be remembered that the origins of the segmental arteries are accessible. In the majority of cases they are easily seen in the hilum and often at points nearer the aorta. This is of practical value, since segmental resection is best carried out from the hilum towards the periphery.

Planning the Area of Resection

It is essential to have a decisive plan of the site and extent of the area to be removed before operation is started, however much this may have to be modified in the heat of the action. The plan is formed mainly on three factors:—

a. Pathology

The arrangement of the renal arterial segments is such that only resection of the upper or lower pole is of practical value, since on anatomical grounds alone, apart from those of pathology, the single resection of, say, the middle or posterior segment would be both impracticable and useless. In practice, the nature of the pathology may necessitate that the site of resection be determined more on the arrangement of the calices, rather than on the arterial pattern alone, and this may call for resection of an arterial segment, with an additional sub-segment from a neighbouring segment. Abeshouse and Lerman (1950) have recorded both personal and collected cases of partial nephrectomy of the upper or lower pole for stone. Of these, there were 107 cases in which the lower pole was removed and 56 cases in which the upper pole was removed; they record that the mid-portion of the kidney (middle calix) was removed in 8 cases. Eberhart and Banks (1952) recorded 15 personal cases in which removal of the upper pole was done in 11 cases and removal of the lower pole in 4 cases. Twinem (1940) found that calculus is more than twice as common in the inferior calix than in the upper one. This fact is most likely to account for the predominance of operation for the removal of the lower pole, rather than the fact that removal of the lower pole is the easier operation to perform.

b. Choosing the Site of Incision

This is rather more difficult than would at first appear, for one's idea on the line of section may seem to be quite clear on viewing the radiographs, but become much more hazy when confronted with a live kidney in the operation field, which has no distinguishing landmarks. I find that the following two manœuvres are very useful: first, examine a number of radiographs, preferably those of an intravenous pyelogram in which the lesion, the calices, and the soft-tissue shadow of the kidney are well shown. It often happens that a composite picture has to be formed, if necessary by superimposition of various films, for not always can good films of both the lesion, the calices, and the soft-tissue shadows of the outline of the kidney be obtained on the same film. Mark the lowest point of the soft-tissue shadow of the kidney on the radiograph (or extreme edge of upper pole, whichever is appropriate), then measure the distance between the point and the upper border of the lesion in the calix to be resected, or the lower border of the lesion in the case of the upper pole. This measurement, and the use of a sterile rule at operation, will give a fairly accurate guide as to the correct site of section, but care must be taken to allow a little leeway on either side. Secondly, at operation use the technique of *serial section.* Bearing in mind that it is always easier to remove a little more kidney tissue if one has underestimated one's line of cut, than to wish afterwards that one had been a little less radical, a series of partial cuts into the renal substance produces a very satisfactory method of determining the exact site of section (*Fig.* 58). Let us say, for example, that a resection is to be done for a stone in a calix, or for a localized tuberculous lesion. The aim of the operation is to remove the lesion, its associated cortex, and to make the actual site of incision through healthy tissue,

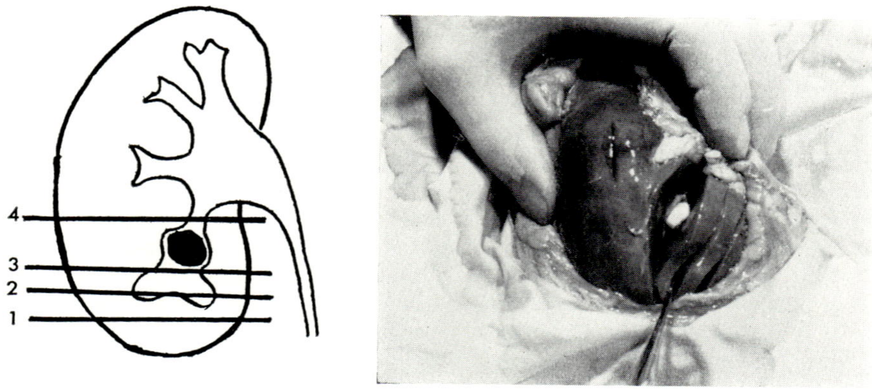

A B

FIG. 58.—Illustrations of the technique of 'serial section'. A, A diagram showing the levels of the consecutive incisions into the kidney, relative to the lesion, which are made in order to find the most suitable site for removal of the diseased segment. The black mass in the lower calix indicates the lesion; sections 1, 2, and 3 are not adequate for they exclude the lesion. Section 4 is satisfactory as it is above the lesion and is made through healthy tissue. In B the process of 'serial section' is shown. The third cut (corresponding to level 3) exposes the lesion, which is a stone in the calix.

taking neither too much nor too little. It is essential to resect through healthy tissue, partly to ensure non-recurrence of disease, and partly to make one's closing sutures through tissue which will heal well. Very few radiographs will tell you where diseased tissue ends and healthy tissue starts. Serial section, however, gives a pretty good guide. Hold the kidney in your hand; decide with the rule where you think the line of section should be. Shorten this by 1 inch, so that the amount of tissue which you propose to remove is *much less than you think it ought to be.* With a knife (not diathermy—do not use diathermy to cut the kidney) make a clean slice down to the level of the calix, but do not extend this slice deeper than the calix. You may perhaps find that you have cut below, or just into the lesion. Make a second slice $\frac{1}{4}$ inch towards the centre of the kidney, that is, nearer your original proposed line. A third and even a fourth slice down to the calix may be necessary until you find that you have cleared the lesion, and are into normal healthy tissue proximal to the site of the disease (*see Fig.* 58). When you have found this, complete the slice by cutting deeper into the kidney tissue, incising through the calix and that posterior part of the pole which is to be removed.

c. The Segmental Arteries

Most of the variations of the segmental arteries of the kidney so far encountered have fallen easily into the groups which have been described, and if at operation dissection is carried from the aorta towards the hilum, the segmental vessels can usually be identified as they originate from the main stem of the renal artery, or from the aorta itself. Knowledge of the variations in the origins of these segmental arteries is important in segmental resection, and no vessel should be ligated until its distribution has been confirmed. For example, it is important to distinguish between Group I and Group II, since ligation of the lower segment artery near its origin would affect only the lower segment in Group I but would leave the middle segment ischaemic in Group II. In the latter group ligation of the lower segment

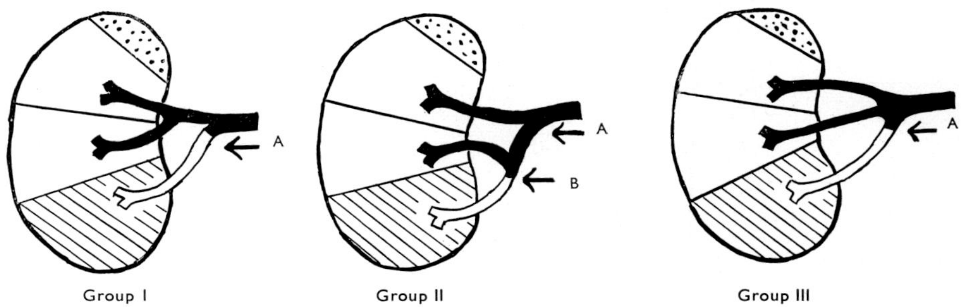

FIG. 59.—The diagram illustrates the importance of determining the arrangement of the anterior segment arteries, *before* ligation of a vessel is made. Ligation of the lower segment artery, at point A, will involve only that segment in kidneys of Groups I and III, but if made at point A in a Group II kidney the middle segment will loose its blood-supply. In resection of the lower segment in Group II, the ligature must be placed at point B.

artery must be made after it has given origin to the middle segment artery, unless it is proposed to remove both middle and lower segments. This is illustrated in *Fig.* 59. If the ligature is made at point A in a Group II kidney, it will affect both the middle and lower segments; hence, if only the lower segment is to be removed, and the kidney belongs to Group II, then the ligature must be applied at point B.

At operation, a temporary compression of a vessel frequently results in a purplish discoloration of the area supplied. This is a useful guide when determining the amount of tissue to be resected (Abeshouse and Lerman, 1950).

A surgeon once told me that on one occasion when he had compressed a segmental artery at operation, the area of the kidney involved had not changed colour as he had expected, and he asked for a possible explanation. I suggested that this failure to change colour might be due to one of three causes; either the surgeon had not compressed the vessel for long enough, or had compressed it incompletely, or the lack of cyanosis might be due to a high oxygen content of the venous blood in the area. In the latter event, the venous blood in the area would continue to flow to some extent, even after the compression of the segmental artery, because there is no segmental arrangement of the intrarenal veins, which have a free anastomosis throughout the entire kidney. This free anastomosis also accounts for some bleeding from the cut surface of the kidney sometimes even after the ligation of the arteries to the area.

The Anatomy of Lower Pole Resection

The anatomical principles of partial nephrectomy in general have already been given; the following notes on the resection of the lower pole in particular may, however, be of use:—

Vessels

Decide whether the arterial arrangement of the kidney falls into that of Group I, II, or III, or whether it has multiple renal arteries. If in Group I or III, seek for the origin of the lower segment artery, establish its distribution by temporary compression, and ligate it. If of Group II, then seek for the origin of the middle segment artery and take care to ligate the lower segment artery at a point after the middle segment vessel has taken its origin, unless, of course, it is proposed to take the middle segment as well. (The middle segment may be small, if the middle calices are small.) Now look on the posterior surface of the kidney for the terminal branches of the posterior segment artery, and if appropriate, ligate these. Remember that the posterior part of the lower pole of the kidney is supplied by the posterior branch of the lower segment artery, that vessel which curls under the neck of the inferior calix, and that this area will be included when the lower segment artery is tied.

If there are multiple renal arteries, these must be identified in the light of the charts given in Chapter Five. The most likely variant in this group is the lower segment artery which arises directly from the aorta, not infrequently passing in front of, and below the pelvi-ureteric junction. Less commonly, its posterior branch may arise from it but outside the kidney substance, and more rarely still from the aorta (*see Fig.* 31, p. 38). If the lower segment artery does arise from the aorta, BEWARE lest the testicular or ovarian artery arises in turn from the lower segment artery, and sometimes quite near the kidney. Ligation of the latter must therefore be made after the artery to the gonad has originated, otherwise testicular atrophy will develop (*see Fig.* 30, p. 36).

Serial Section

This has already been described. Care must be taken when making the half-slice down as far as the calix not to deepen this cut too readily without being prepared to deal with the haemorrhage which may occur from the posterior branch of the lower segment artery as it curls round under the neck of the calix. This is not likely to trap the surgeon who has ligated the segmental artery, or has a clamp across the renal pedicle, in advance, but it can be a potent source of bleeding for one who is not forewarned.

Lastly, when the serial section of choice has been made, take care when completing the cut through the posterior part of the kidney not to cut into the pelvis. It is not difficult to make this mistake, only to find that one has an extensive incision in the pelvis to suture, in addition to closing the calix. An accidental incision such as this increases the risk of urinary fistula.

Haemostasis on the Cut Surface

This I do by meticulous ligation of every bleeding vessel by a 'figure-of-eight' stitch, placed so that when the knot is tied, the catgut pulls through the soft tissue of the cortex and the vessel is caught in the noose (*see Fig.* 71, p. 86).

Secondly, equal care is taken in the closure of the calicine stump or stumps. This is done by a 3/0 atraumatic catgut continuous suture, but knotted at intervals. It must be remembered that *around the calix is a very extensive plexus of veins*, and often it is from these veins rather than the arteries that the postoperative bleeding arises. A careful closure of the calix will often deal with much of the venous bleeding. On looking at the casts of the intrarenal arteries, as shown in earlier chapters, it may be a little difficult to visualize how they may appear when viewed in horizontal section. I have therefore made a fresh set of casts, subsequently

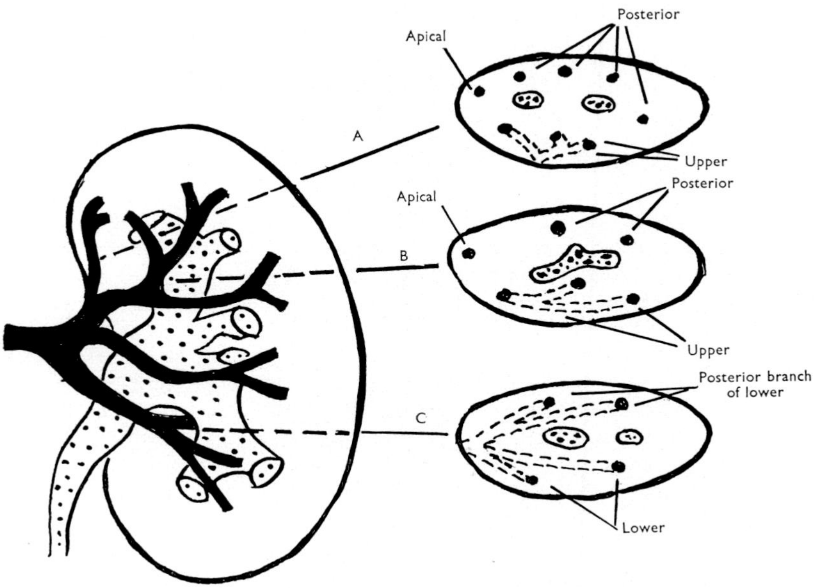

FIG. 60.—A diagram indicating the position of the branches of the segmental arteries which will be encountered on the cut, horizontal surface of the kidney, during the operation of partial nephrectomy. Control of these is made by 'figure-of-eight' sutures. A and B indicate sites of resection for the upper pole, whereas C is for the lower pole. Note that the incision at B MUST BE above the level of the posterior division.

embedded one in a block of resin, and then cut through the whole in serial sections, on a horizontal plane, so as to make this presentation of the vessels more clear (*Fig.* 60).

Arteries seen on Horizontal Section

On viewing the cut surface of the remaining portion of the kidney, when the lower pole has been removed, the following structures will be seen from before, backwards. Near the anterior surface of the organ will be at least two branches of the lower segment artery, one on the medial and one on the lateral side. Behind these will be the inferior calix, and behind this, in turn, will be the posterior branch of the lower segment artery, presenting probably as two small, divided vessels. These are illustrated at level C in *Fig.* 60. If, however, the section through the kidney is made at a lower level than that of level C, the number of divided vessels will be more numerous, though smaller in calibre. Likewise, the inferior calix may be replaced by two minor calices.

Closure of the Kidney

In contrast to some authors, I do not make flaps of cortical tissue in order to close the raw surface of the kidney. I advocate a clean guillotine or horizontal cut, straight through the kidney, from front to back. I am against the making of flaps on a number of grounds; in the making of flaps, cortex may be left behind which is close to the disease process, and would better have been removed. Alternatively, if the cortical tissue is healthy, then, by utilizing it for the making of the flaps, it is being needlessly sacrificed. Also, flaps of tissue will have little or no blood-supply (especially if catgut sutures are placed through them, in order to 'turn the flaps inwards'), and this will lead inevitably to infection or ischaemia, and likewise hide a haematoma.

The Anatomy of Upper Pole Resection

Resection of the upper pole will involve removal of the apical segment, and since this usually contains such a small portion of the upper calix, it will be necessary to remove sub-segments of the upper and posterior segments as well.

Vessels

Depending on the size of the upper calix and the lesion, it may be necessary to ligate the upper segment artery at its origin, so that both its apical and horizontal branches are involved in the ensuing haemostasis, or it may be better to divide and ligate only the apical branch, which runs towards the upper pole. This will almost certainly have to be picked up within the substance of the kidney, as the serial section cuts down on to it. The artery to the apical segment must be sought and ligated. It may arise in the hilum from the upper segment artery (Type I) or from the junction of the anterior and posterior divisions (Type II) (*see Fig.* 6, p. 9). It may arise from the posterior division (Type IV) or it may arise from nearer the aorta (Type III) and appear as an 'aberrant' or multiple renal artery.

If of this latter group of variants, then those of IIIc and IIId (*see Fig.* 28, p. 35) are of the most importance; in variant IIIc, the artery to the apical segment breaks into a leash of vessels, each of which enters the segment separately; if of variant IIId, the inferior artery to the suprarenal arises from the segmental artery, so that the latter must be ligated after the suprarenal vessel has originated from it. Watch also for the unusually early origin of the posterior division from the aorta (*see Fig.* 27, p. 34), and do not ligate it in the belief that it is the artery to the apical segment. Its size is distinctive.

Serial Section

It is very important that when the final line of section is made, that this is *above* the curve of the artery to the posterior segment, which passes behind and in close association with the junction of the pelvis and the upper calix (*see Figs.* 5B, 8B, and 13B, pp. 9, 10, and 15). Accidental damage to this vessel will result in very considerable haemorrhage, and its subsequent ligation will involve a very large area on the posterior surface of the kidney, in perpetual infarction.

Haemostasis

In principle as for the lower pole.

Arteries seen on Horizontal Section

On viewing the remaining portion of the kidney, when the upper pole is removed, the mouths of the arteries presenting on the cut surface will vary to some extent in size and number depending upon the level of section, although the actual segmental arteries involved will be the same (*see Fig.* 60). At level A, from before backwards, the arteries will be the apical branches of the upper segment artery, probably two or three in number. To the medial side of these will be the apical segment artery. In the centre of the cut surface will be two minor upper calices, and behind these, the apical branches of the posterior segment artery, probably three or four in number.

If the serial section is made at a lower level, say at level B, then in addition to two mouths of the apical branch of the upper segment artery, there may also be a branch of the horizontal branch of the upper segment artery lying more to the lateral edge. On the posterior side, the branches of the posterior segment artery will probably be fewer, but larger in calibre. One other point to remember is that if the apical segment artery is small, as it arises from the anterior division, or alternatively is of Type III, then there may be two smaller apical arteries on the medial side of the cut surface, instead of one larger one.

Closure of the Kidney

In principle as for the lower pole.

Anatomy of Resection of Mid-zone

In general I do not view with much enthusiasm operations for resection of the middle zone of the kidney, mainly because neither the anatomy of the calices nor the arterial systems of this area lend themselves to satisfactory resection nor reconstitution.

A wedge resection of the middle of the kidney is possible, however, but is only suitable for peripheral lesions, such as old scars, cortical abscesses, and so on. If a wedge resection is done, then the arterial vessels must be controlled by ligature sutures on the cut surface, for no attempt at segmental ligation is possible. Also it is the veins on the cut surface which are the most troublesome to control.

Large cysts, on the lateral surface of the kidney are, I find, best excised. Removal of the portion within the kidney is easy. It often 'shells out', but the control of the gentle but continuous venous bleeding from the raw surface is quite another matter. In view of this, it is often safer to leave undisturbed that small patch of the cyst wall which is embedded in the substance of the kidney.

Removal of Staghorn Calculus

In view of the anatomical demonstration in previous chapters that Brodel's line is by no means a bloodless area, both from the viewpoint of the arterial supply and also the very extensive venous system, it was necessary to devise a method of removing very large, or staghorn, calculi from the kidney, by some method other than that of splitting the kidney along its lateral border.

This can be achieved quite satisfactorily by a partial nephrectomy, removing either the upper or lower pole of the kidney, depending on the size and shape of the stone. The following description and diagrams illustrate my own technique.

Single Staghorn

The single horn, as shown in *Fig.* 53 (p. 57) is easily removed together with the calix which contains it, by an upper pole resection.

Small Staghorn

Fig. 61A shows a small staghorn calculus whose main bulk lies in the lowest calix, there being only small stumps in the middle and upper calices. The following procedure is carried out:—

First Stage

The lower pole of the kidney is resected. This automatically opens the lower calix and also the lower border of the pelvis, thus giving a far greater mobility to the stone than is afforded by a simple pyelotomy.

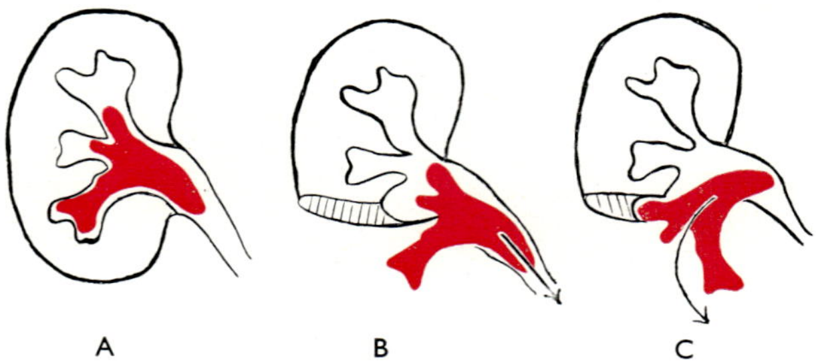

FIG. 61.—A diagram of the stages of removal of a small staghorn calculus (A) whose main bulk lies in the inferior calix. In B the lower pole of the kidney has been removed; the inferior horn of the stone is no longer anchored by the kidney substance, and is now pushed downwards towards the pelvi-ureteric junction. This action frees the middle and upper horns from their calices, so that in the third stage (C), the calculus is rotated downwards and medially and is removed, upside down, in one piece.

Second Stage (*Fig.* 61B)

The stone is now pushed downwards towards the pelvi-ureteric junction; this action in turn frees the middle and upper horns of the stone from their calices.

Third Stage (*Fig.* 61C)

The calculus is then rotated downwards and medially and is removed upside down in one piece.

Moderate-size Staghorn

Fig. 62A shows a staghorn calculus in which the largest part occupies the upper calix, although there are quite large 'stumps' in the middle and lower calices. I advocate the following technique:—

First Stage

Resect the upper pole of the kidney exposing the upper part of the stone.

Second Stage (*Fig.* 62B)

The stone now is mobilized sufficiently for it to be pushed down towards the pelvi-ureteric junction. This movement in turn frees the stumps from their respective middle and lower calices.

Third Stage

The upper part of the calculus is now rotated upwards and medially. This movement at the same time disengages the lower part of the stone (*Fig.* 62C) from the

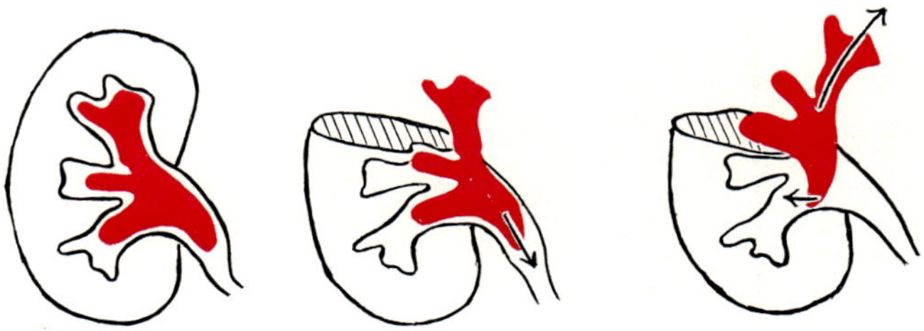

FIG. 62.—A diagram of the stages of removal of a staghorn calculus of medium size (A), whose largest part lies in the upper calix. The upper pole of the kidney is first resected, so that the upper horn of the stone is no longer anchored (B) by the kidney substance. The calculus is now free to be pushed down towards the pelvi-ureteric junction, thus freeing the middle and lower horns of the stone. Finally, the upper part of the calculus is rotated upwards and medially (C), this movement at the same time disengages the lower part of the stone from the pelvis, so that the whole stone is moved about a fulcrum as it is withdrawn from the kidney.

pelvis and moves it horizontally, thus enabling the whole calculus to be moved like a lever about a fulcrum and finally withdrawn from the kidney.

Large Staghorn Kidney

Fig. 63A illustrates a calculus with large horns in each of the three major calices. The operative procedure is this:—

First Stage

The upper pole of the kidney is resected, thereby exposing the upper part of the stone, and at the same time opening the upper part of the pelvi-calicine system. The upper horn of the stone is then gently retracted medially, so that the shaft of the horn entering the middle calix is then exposed.

Second Stage (*Fig.* 63B)

The middle horn is then deliberately fractured at point A as marked on the diagram. To do this I hold the kidney in my left hand; *this is important in order that the shock waves of the 'osteotomy' are absorbed and not disseminated through the kidney substance.* With my right hand I then hold a small osteotome at the point A on the stone. An assistant then gives a gentle tap with a mallet on the osteotome and the middle horn is severed. I prefer this method to that of using bone forceps; the latter tend to crush the stone, which often breaks up into a number of fragments. These are not only more difficult to remove, but small flakes tend to get left behind and these will form nuclei for fresh stones. An 'osteotomy' on the other hand gives a clean cut, and so enables the separated stone to be removed in one piece.

Third Stage

The upper horn of the calculus is retracted further in a medial direction, to expose, and partly withdraw, the shaft of the lower horn from its calix. This also is fractured by 'osteotomy' at point B.

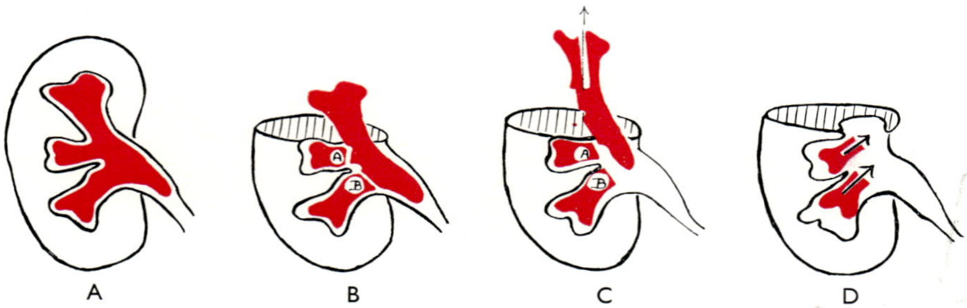

FIG. 63.—A diagram illustrating the stages of removal of a large staghorn calculus (A), with big horns in all calices. The upper pole of the kidney is first resected. The calculus, now no longer anchored by the kidney tissue of the upper pole (B), is retracted medially, so as to expose the neck of the horn in the middle calix, which is fractured with a small osteotome at point A. This exposes the neck of the inferior horn, which is fractured in like manner at point B. The upper horn and pelvic part of the stone is now free to be removed in an upward direction through the open upper calix as shown in C. Finally, the middle and lower horns of the stone, which are now free in their calices (D), are each removed through the open upper pole.

Fourth Stage (*Fig.* 63C)

The upper horn, together with the pelvic component is now drawn upwards and removed.

Fifth Stage (*Fig.* 63D)

The middle and lower horns, which are now loose in their sockets, are each removed through the open upper pole of the kidney.

CHAPTER EIGHT

RENAL HYPOTHERMIA: AN AID TO PARTIAL NEPHRECTOMY

THE discovery of the segmental arrangement of the intrarenal arteries laid an anatomical foundation for segmental resection of the kidney. As the study of these vessels proceeded however, it became apparent that, if resection of renal tissue was to be done with meticulous technique similar to that used in the resection of lung tissue, then a considerable amount of time would be necessary for the operation. There is no doubt that careful resection, haemostasis, and closure of the calicine stump is essential to prevent the postoperative complications of haemorrhage and fistula. This therefore necessitates an operation in a bloodless field by occlusion of the renal artery.

The kidney, however, is an organ with complex biochemical functions and, like the brain, though to a lesser extent, will not withstand loss of its blood-supply and the accompanying anoxia for any great length of time without possible impairment of some of its function.

The idea occurred to me that if the cells of the renal cortex could be induced into a state of temporary hibernation by cooling, similar to that achieved by the brain in cardiac surgery, the biochemical disturbances produced by anoxia of renal tissue by prolonged clamping of the renal artery might also be reduced and thereby give the surgeon more time in which to perform the resection. The prospect seemed feasible and, moreover, since the kidney presented an insular circulation, the need to cool the whole body seemed unnecessary.

Whilst on a visit to his Clinic, I found that Professor Carl Semb of Oslo had had a similar idea and that he had carried out animal investigations and preliminary surgical experiments. The surgical technique described here is based upon that of Semb (1956), but has modifications.

RATIONALE

Postoperative disturbance of renal function may result from: (*a*) handling the kidney; (*b*) compression of the renal artery. The process of mobilization of the kidney, particularly if the organ has a short pedicle or is adherent, may produce a disturbance of function in the postoperative period. This may be complete failure of the kidney to excrete, together with electrolyte imbalance or, if less severely affected, merely a diminution in the quantity and quality of urine. Experimental compression of the renal pedicle in dogs for 3 hours gave some degree of nitrogen retention for 3 days but function returned to normal in 3 weeks (Van Slyke, Phillips, Hamilton, Archibald, Dole, and Emerson, 1944). In man, clamping of the renal pedicle for 50 minutes (Semb, 1956) was followed by severe impairment of filtration and tubular reabsorption, but recovery was complete in 6 weeks. Clamping the renal artery in man for 18 minutes produced moderate temporary impairment, whilst occlusion for 10–12 minutes gave only a mild reaction.

This shows that the renal function is likely to be impaired to some extent if the artery is occluded for more than 12 minutes, and that this disturbance may be further increased if the mobilization dissection has been difficult—a finding not uncommon in the diseased kidney, particularly one selected for partial nephrectomy. In practice it is seldom possible to perform a partial nephrectomy with a technique sufficiently meticulous to ensure freedom from postoperative sequelae, in the space of 12 minutes. Can, therefore, these disturbances of metabolic and excretory function which follow prolonged occlusion of the renal artery be reduced by subjecting the renal cortex to hypothermia?

Experimental Hypothermia in Dogs

A nephrectomy was done in a number of healthy dogs (Birkeland, Vogt, Krog, and Semb, 1956). Subsequently the artery to the remaining kidney was occluded for periods varying up to 8 hours, and during this time the kidney only was cooled to temperatures varying from 0° C. to 37° C. The results showed that those dogs whose kidneys had been cooled to 5–10° C., survived even when their renal vessels had been clamped for as long as 7 hours, whereas those not subjected to hypothermia died after 3 hours' renal occlusion.

PREOPERATIVE INVESTIGATION

In addition to the clinical and urological investigations (which include an intravenous pyelogram and full laboratory examination of the urine), a number of more elaborate investigations are done, not only to establish the function of each kidney but also to provide an additional check as to the extent of the disease. This information is provided by serum biochemistry and bilateral ureteric catheterization. The latter yields: (1) Microscopy of urine deposit, reaction, culture, and sensitivity of organisms from each kidney; (2) Divided renal function tests; (3) Bilateral retrograde pyelograms.

Ureteric Catheterization

Apart from local urethral anaesthetic in the male, ureteric catheterization is done *without anaesthetic* and *without premedication.* This is important. General anaesthesia and even premedication will produce a considerable reduction in renal excretion and so make the investigation of little use. Further, the customary period of 4 hours' preoperative starvation reduces the urine flow still more. Patients are therefore encouraged to eat and drink right up to the moment of leaving the ward for the theatre.

A large whistle-tipped catheter has produced the most satisfactory results. The multiple-eyed catheters used by Semb for lower ureteric catheterization have not been found to give any advantage over the standard type, particularly as small volumes of urine only are needed for modern biochemical techniques. In general, the first 2 or 3 ml. of urine from each kidney are collected in separate bottles for bacteriological investigation, and the next 7 ml. from each side in chemically clean tubes are taken for the full range of divided renal function tests. At the same time 7 ml. of blood are taken from a vein.

On an average the process takes about 20 minutes, including cystoscopy, after which the patient proceeds to pyelography. The patient returns home after 48 hours to await the result of the function tests. This saves much tedious waiting for both patients and staff and reduces the blockage of beds. The patient is readmitted at a later date for operation.

Biochemical Investigations

In cases of calculous disease serum calcium, phosphorus, and alkaline phosphatase estimations are done for evidence of the possible presence of a parathyroid tumour. In all cases the following investigations are done:—

Serum:
- Urea
- Creatinine
- Inorganic phosphate
- Sodium
- Potassium
- Chloride

Urine (from right and left kidneys):
- Volume (ml.)
- Volume per min. (ml.)
- Urea (mg. per 100 ml.)
- Creatinine (mg. per 100 ml.)
- Inorganic phosphate
- Sodium
- Potassium
- Chloride

From these are calculated the following:—

Tubular reabsorption of (from right and left kidneys):
- Water
- Sodium
- Urea
- Potassium
- Chloride

Final Assessment of Renal Function

Assessment is made on the divided renal function tests and on the intravenous pyelogram. There is no doubt that the intravenous pyelogram is a most valuable guide to renal function. There are pitfalls of which to beware. A kidney from which the excretion is fast and in which peristalsis is brisk may show little evidence of dye compared with its fellow. Likewise a relatively functionless lower pole may appear to have good function purely because the dye has collected in its 'sump' by gravity.

In general, biochemical assessment of function is grouped under three degrees: normal, moderate, and poor. It is important to determine the function of the 'bad' kidney by comparison with that of its fellow, rather than with the results obtained in other patients. In these investigations the biochemist was not told which was the 'bad' kidney, so that an independent assessment was made. In general, function is assessed on the ability to reabsorb water and sodium. 'If the excretion of water is within normal limits (not exceeding 2 per cent) severe damage to the kidney may be ruled out. If simultaneously with a low concentration of endogenous creatinine the concentration of sodium in urine is higher than in plasma, it may be assumed that the higher excretion of water is not caused by severe damage to the kidney' (Schück, Hradic, Fabicen, and Svobodova, 1960).

For example, one of our cases gave these figures. The right kidney showed 6·7 per cent water excretion, but the urine sodium was 37 mEq./l., compared with a serum sodium of 139 mEq./l., thus ruling out an osmotic diuresis and indicating a severe damage to the kidney. The left kidney, on the other hand, showed a water excretion of 2·7 per cent but in this case urine sodium was 135 mEq./l., indicating an increased water excretion as the result of an osmotic diuresis.

Aortography

Routine aortography was not done. In those cases where additional information was needed concerning the nature of the blood-supply to a particular part of the kidney, as, for instance, a suspected area of avascularity in the renal cortex in a case of hypertension, an aortogram was done by the Seldinger technique.

THEATRE EQUIPMENT

Care was taken to ensure that the equipment was simple for three reasons: first, finance; secondly, complicated equipment tends to 'go wrong' and often needs frequent maintenance which is not always easy to obtain at short notice; thirdly, complicated equipment necessitates trained assistants who are not always available in the smaller hospitals. The essential equipment consists of:—

2 Needle-thermocouples
2 Thermocouples for insertion into the mouth
Temperature measuring equipment matched to the thermocouples
A plastic bag which can be sterilized
Cooling medium
Occlusion clamp for the renal artery

Temperature Measuring Equipment and Thermocouples

My own equipment consists of a Cambridge Skin Temperature Measuring Outfit made by the Cambridge Instrument Company. This is accurate, easy to use, easy to calibrate, and portable. The needle-thermocouples are contained in a standard 1-mm. needle, but with a very small head and with surgical plastic covering of the connecting leads sealed over the head of the needle so that the whole unit can be sterilized. The thermocouples for insertion into the mouth consist of 28-gauge thermocouple wire with the junction cemented to the end of the surgical plastic, with an overall diameter of $\frac{1}{8}$ inch. The length of the leads for all thermocouples is about 6 or 7 feet. This is important to prevent crowding round the theatre table. All thermocouples are matched so that readings can be taken in rapid succession from any one of them.

Plastic Bag

I use a simple polythene bag of good quality as sold for domestic use. A small hole is cut in the centre of the bottom of the bag and to this is attached a length of glass tubing. The tubing is $\frac{1}{2}$ inch in diameter and about 3 inches long. The bag is bound to the tubing by Mersalene, and the joint is watertight. It is advisable to have two or three bags available as spares.

Cooling Medium

Cracked ice can be used (Semb, personal communication). I do not find this very satisfactory for it is difficult to get solid ice out of bottles of sterile water which have been frozen, the ice is difficult to handle, and theatre sterility tends to be impaired. One morning in November, my wife reminded me to place antifreeze in the radiator of the car. This gave me an idea and so I applied to the problem the same notion of using 'antifreeze'. This worked well. A solution of 30 per cent glycerin in water is prepared by the hospital pharmacy and sterilized in bottles ready for use. A number of these are stored in the cold compartment of a laboratory refrigerator at a temperature of about $-3°$ C. The solution remains fluid and soon warms up to 2° C. on being taken to the theatre a few minutes before being required.

Occlusion Clamp

Although experiments were made with a view to using a pneumatic clamp, in the end a satisfactory occlusion, without apparent damage to the renal pedicle, was obtained by the use of a curved-on-flat intestinal clamp, the blades of which are covered with protecting pads of vinyl sponge. These are made in the hospital and are changed for each case.

Sterilization of Equipment

The needle-thermocouples and mouth-thermocouples are stored and sterilized in dry-formalin fumes. The plastic bags are sterilized in Roccal solution for the 24 hours prior to operation; care should be taken when packing the plastic bags in the sterilizing solution to ensure that no air bubbles collect or else sterilization may not be adequate. Sterilization of the cooling fluid is done in an autoclave as for intravenous fluids.

THE OPERATION

Equipment

The Cambridge Skin Temperature Measuring Outfit is placed in the theatre suite overnight in order to take up room temperature.

Anaesthesia

A standard anaesthetic with use of relaxants is given. Blood-pressure readings are taken.

Position of Patient

This is important, for much of the ease of access and exposure of the kidney may depend on positioning. The patient is placed in the lateral position. It is better and safer to open up the renal angle by 'breaking the table' than by use of the kidney bridge. An intravenous drip is set up. An anaesthetic screen is placed in position: this has an additional use, as the sterile thermocouples can be stored in a sterile rubber diathermy scabbard attached to the screen after towelling. They are then easily available and out of harm's way.

Calibration of Temperature Measuring Outfit

The assistant responsible for recording temperatures sets up his apparatus near the anaesthetist and preferably behind the surgeon. One sterile needle-thermocouple and one sterile mouth-thermocouple are kept in the scabbard and the leads connected; the other mouth-thermocouple is handed to the anaesthetist who places its tip in the oropharynx of the patient. It is also connected. These three thermocouples will be used to record the temperature of the kidney, cooling fluid, and body temperatures respectively. Calibration of the box is carried out by the assistant during the towelling and the early part of the operation.

Incision

An oblique incision is made. It courses along the twelfth rib, but in patients who are big or obese, it is made along the line of the eleventh rib. The muscle is cut with diathermy. The twelfth rib is often resected and in obese patients sometimes the eleventh rib as well.

Exposure of the Kidney

After incision of the lumbodorsal fascia, the fascia of Zuckerkandl is incised. I take pains to preserve this fascia and emphasize that the fascia is incised and not torn by blunt or finger dissection. The wound is then held by a self-retaining retractor. The kidney is mobilized and this is done with scissor dissection, handling being reduced to a minimum. As the dissection is carried round the poles, especially on the medial side, watch should be kept for the presence of segmental arteries which may be making an extrahilar entry to their segments (the so-called 'aberrant arteries'). The renal pedicle is then also mobilized and cleared gently, but 'stripping' must be avoided. Examination is now made for any evidence of the group of the anterior segment vessels at the hilum.

Occlusion of the Renal Artery and Application of the Plastic Bag (*Fig.* 64)

Before the bag is applied preliminary tests are made with both thermocouples (*Fig.* 65). It is wise to have one spare needle-thermocouple sterilized in case of

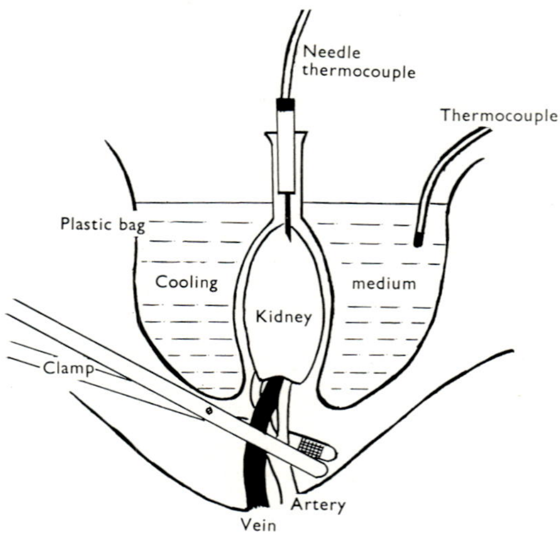

FIG. 64.—A diagram showing the plastic bag, cooling medium, and thermocouples, in position around the kidney. The arterial occlusion clamp compresses the renal pedicle.

emergency. The plastic bag is taken and placed round the kidney so that the small glass tube projects upwards from the surface of the kidney (*Fig*. 66). The lower

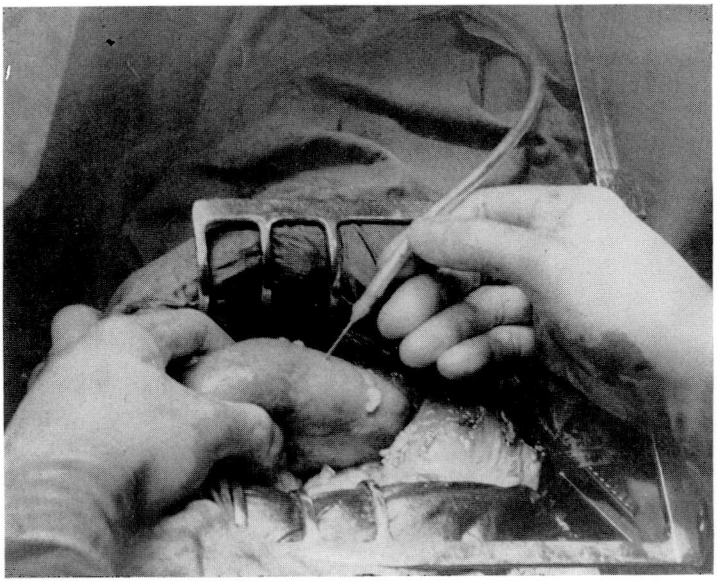

FIG. 65.—The kidney is exposed and a preliminary test is made to check the activity of the thermocouple.

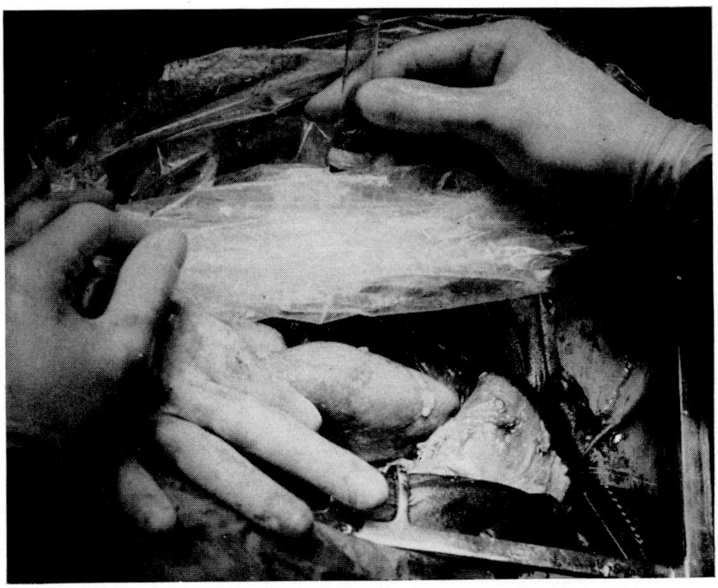

FIG. 66.—The plastic bag is opened out preparatory to enveloping the kidney.

folds of the bag are held close to the renal pedicle by a sterile rubber band which is slipped over the whole kidney. A trial application is now made to see from which angle (*Fig.* 67) the occlusion clamp can be most easily and comfortably applied to the renal artery. Having done this, the clamp is left in position but is not closed.

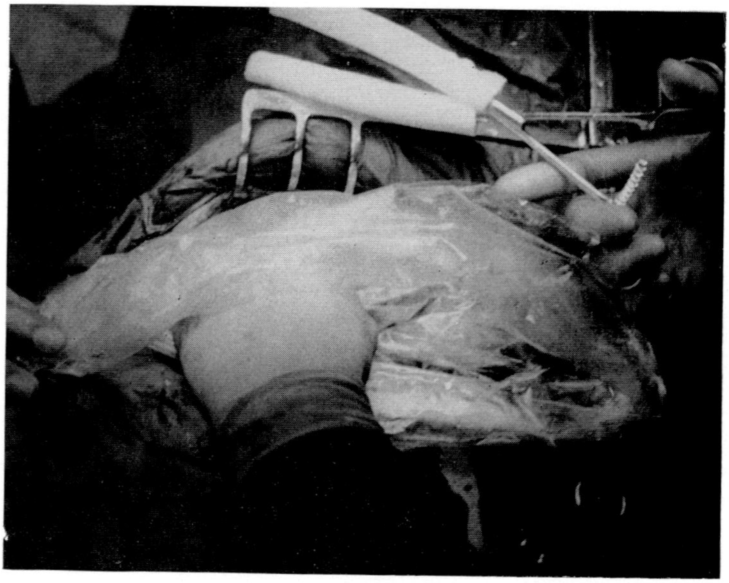

FIG. 67.—The plastic bag is now in position around the kidney, to which it is held by an elastic band in the depths of the bag adjacent to the pedicle. The arterial occlusion clamp, with its protecting pads, is about to be placed across the renal pedicle.

Cooling the Kidney

The sterile cooling fluid is now poured into the plastic bag (*Fig.* 68) and its temperature recorded by the sterile mouth-thermocouple from the scabbard. The needle-thermocouple is placed down the small glass tube so that its tip enters the cortex of the kidney to a depth of 2 or 3 mm. It is essential that *the needle shall not be placed too far into the kidney substance*, for the cooling process is confined to the *surface layers of the cortex*. If the needle is placed too deep, then false readings and over-cooling may result. The occlusion clamp is closed. Temperature readings are taken of the renal cortex every half-minute (*Fig.* 69). In practice I find that a satisfactory drop in temperature with adequate after-cooling is achieved in about 4–5 minutes, the temperature falling from 37° C. to 21° C., though occasionally it may fall to 17° C. in this time. Too rapid cooling is best avoided, for it may do some damage to the superficial cortical layers and after-cooling will not be so well maintained when the bag is removed.

Resection of Renal Tissue

The cooling fluid is sucked away and the bag removed; the occlusion clamp remains closed. The kidney will feel cold to the touch. The site of section is now determined. I find it helpful to measure in centimetres a suitable site on the pyelogram films from one or other pole of the kidney and then at operation to apply this, using a sterile rule. A curved incision is made in the capsule of the kidney only, and if possible it is separated from the underlying cortex and turned back as two flaps to the site of the proposed line of section. The kidney substance is

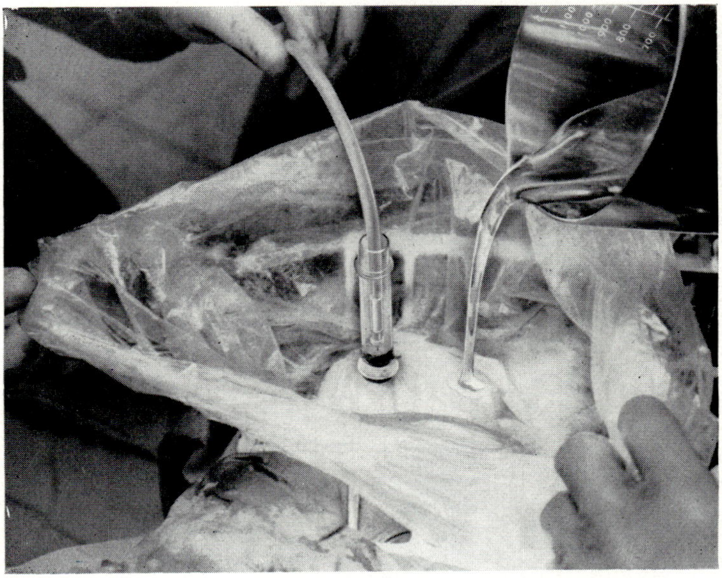

FIG. 68.—The cooling medium (with 'antifreeze') is poured into the plastic bag. The needle-thermocouple is in position inside the glass tube which protects it from the cooling fluid. Note that only a few mm. of the needle are inserted into the renal cortex.

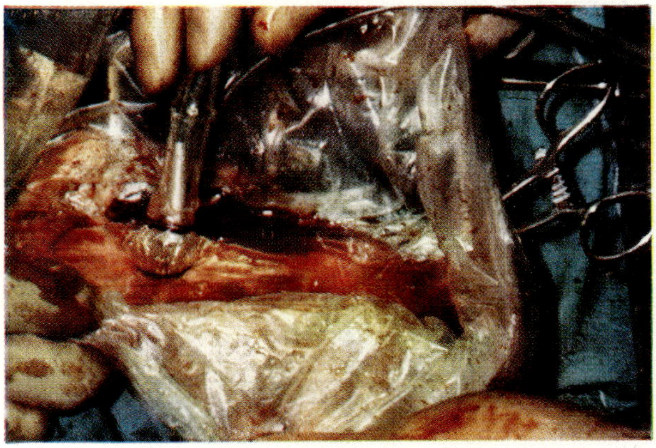

FIG. 69.—A photograph in colour of the process of cooling the kidney, during the operation of partial nephrectomy. The cooling fluid is held around the kidney by a plastic bag for about 4 minutes; the temperature of the renal cortex falls from 37° C. to 21° C.

incised with a knife, through a point a little distal to the intended line of resection; the cut is carried straight down to the calix which is distinguished from the surrounding tissue by its whiteness. If this line of section is not correct, when, for example, the focus of disease is not adequately included in the portion to be resected, then further cuts are made until a suitable plane is found (*Fig.* 70). The calix is divided separately so as to leave a small stump of normal calicine tissue for subsequent closure.

Haemostasis and Closure of Calicine Stump

Haemostasis and closure of the calicine stump must be meticulous. If it has been possible to isolate and ligate the segmental arteries which supply the portion to be

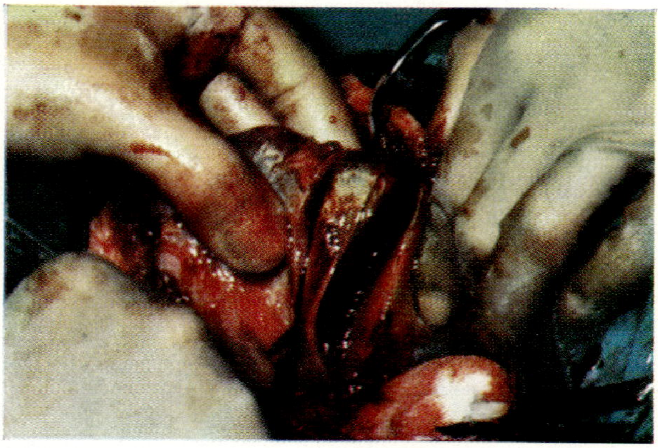

FIG. 70.—A photograph taken during operation of partial nephrectomy, after the application of local hypothermia. 'Serial section' is being carried out in order to determine the correct point of resection of the diseased segment. The arterial occlusion clamp is in the foreground.

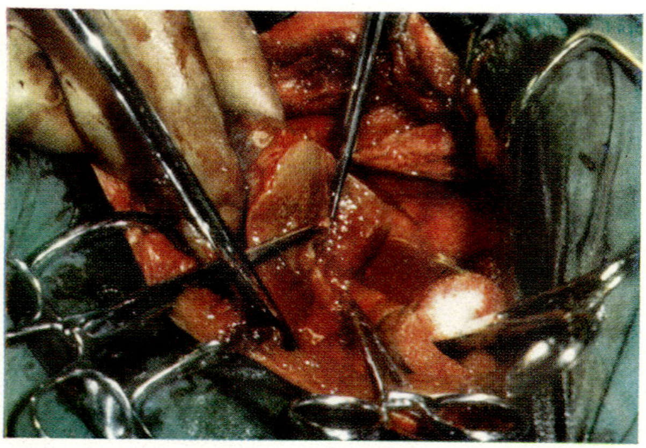

FIG. 71.—The diseased portion of the kidney has been removed, and the photograph shows the cut horizontal surface of the remainder of the kidney. Mosquito-forceps grasp the mouths of the branches of the lower segment artery, which have been divided in the process of resection. (See also *Fig.* 60.)

resected, much of the haemostasis will have been achieved already. If not, the divided intrarenal arteries must be picked up with curved mosquito-forceps in the renal substance (*Fig.* 71). Knowledge of the anatomy of the intrarenal arteries enables one to judge with accuracy where these divided vessels will be in any one plane of section. Simple ligature of these vessels on the cut surface is not satisfactory; I prefer to do a 'figure-of-eight' stitch: it is simple and quick, and seldom

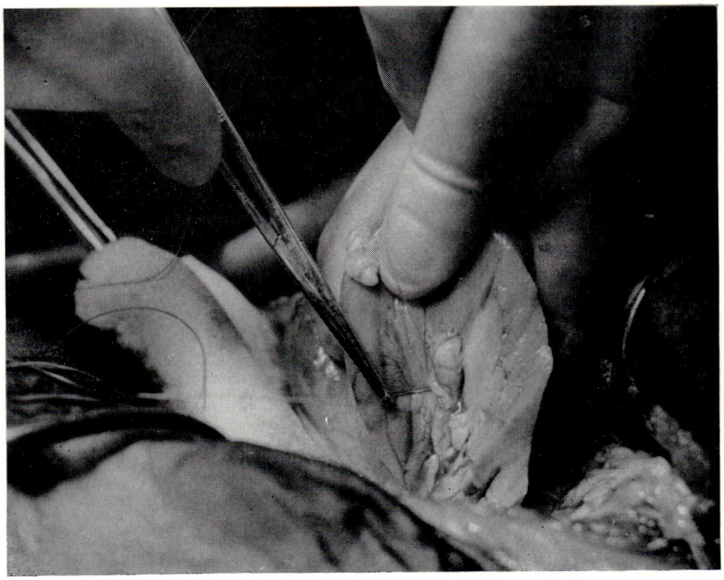

FIG. 72.—Closure of the calicine stump. The arterial occlusion clamp on the left remains closed until haemostasis is complete.

tears out. A large calix is closed by a continuous mattress stitch (*Fig.* 72), and oversewn; a small calix is closed by a single continuous suture. I use 3/0 plain catgut with a 20-mm. atraumatic half-circle needle. There is a hazard for which one should watch. Occasionally on the cut surface of the kidney one may see a wide-mouthed vessel which is not part of the calicine system and may not bleed. It is probably a main renal vein which may have direct communication with the inferior vena cava. Commonly there is a single vein, but sometimes there may be as many as four veins, some of which enter the poles of the kidney individually. Such divided veins on the cut surface must be closed, or else profuse bleeding may result when the occlusion clamp is removed.

Completion of the Operation

The occlusion clamp is removed. This ends the period of 'resection time', the average time of which is 18 minutes (*Fig.* 73). Haemostasis is checked. The temperature of the kidney is recorded again and it will be found usually to have returned to normal or a few degrees below normal. If flaps of capsule are available they are placed over the cut surface of the kidney and sutured in position without tension. In contrast to Semb (1955) I do not suture the kidney substance for I believe that the tension caused thereby, and the practice of making 'flaps' of renal substance in order to effect such closure, may possibly lead to future ischaemia of those flaps, and maybe to eventual hypertension.

Closure of the Wound

The kidney is replaced in its bed and the fascia of Zuckerkandl, which has been carefully preserved, is sutured so as to retain the kidney in its position and thereby reduce possible torsion. The renal bed is drained.

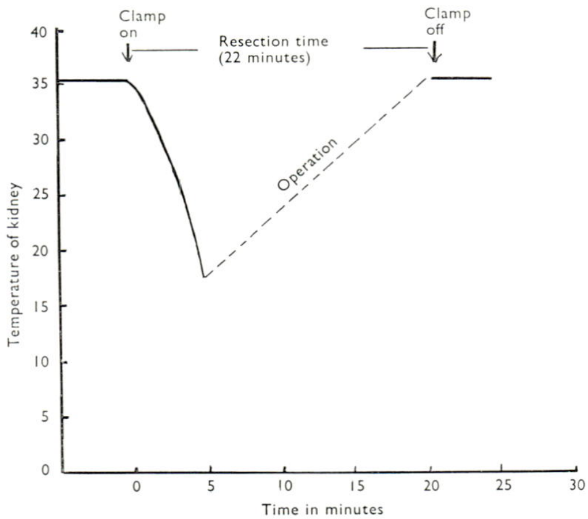

FIG. 73.—A graph showing the temperature of the kidney during the process of cooling and at the end of partial nephrectomy.

POSTOPERATIVE CARE

The intravenous drip is kept running for 24–36 hours, mainly to promote urine formation and so reduce clot formation and colic. An antibiotic is given for 4 or 5 days. During the first 3 days a blood-urea estimation is done twice daily and serum electrolytes once a day. Early mobilization of the patient is encouraged. The majority of patients are up and about by the sixth day and are home soon after the tenth postoperative day.

COMMENT ON THE PHYSIOLOGY OF HYPOTHERMIA TECHNIQUE

Estimation of the value of this technique has been made from both clinical and biochemical aspects. From the clinical point of view the general well-being of the patient, even in the immediate postoperative period, has been remarkable. Urine flow was good, with minimal haematuria which cleared within 24–48 hours. Two patients (1 of whom was a diabetic weighing 18 stone) upon whom operation was done on the only kidney which showed evidence of adequate function gave urine outputs of 2520 ml. and 2110 ml. respectively, with normal or slightly increased concentration in the first 24 hours after operation. Blood-urea, in general, was little changed, and in some cases even dropped below the preoperative level on the second or third postoperative day. Hamilton Stewart (1960) also reported no ill-effects in 41 cases of partial nephrectomy under local hypothermia.

Assessment from the biochemical aspect in each case has been more difficult owing to the technical difficulty of collecting urine from both ureters during the operation, for the catheters tend to become blocked with blood, pus, or debris. Two sets of information, however, have been obtained.

First, the behaviour of the 'other kidney'—that is, a normal kidney was investigated during the operation on its fellow. Urine was collected from a ureteric

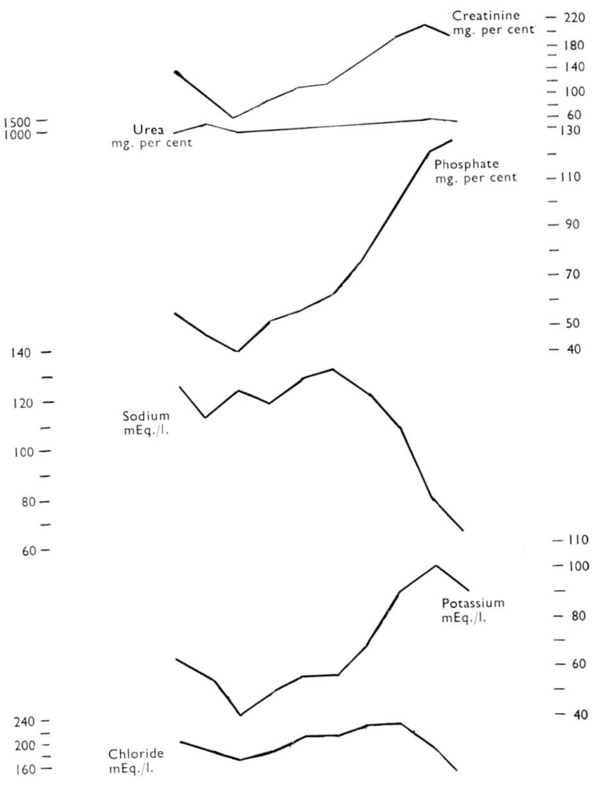

FIG. 74.—A graph of urine analysis from the 'other kidney' during operation on its fellow. Urea output and blood-urea were constant. Potassium, phosphate, and creatinine excretions were increased, but there was some retention of chlorides and sodium.

catheter throughout the operation, during which the blood-pressure was reasonably constant. Blood and urine analyses showed that during the operation, urea output and blood-urea remained constant; the potassium, phosphate, and creatinine excretions were increased, but in contrast to these there was some retention of chlorides and sodium (*Fig.* 74).

Secondly, an attempt was made to find out how soon function would re-start in the kidney subjected to cooling and partial nephrectomy, and to compare its excretion with its fellow. The figures were obtained from blood and urine analyses (*Fig.* 75) during the operation upon a patient, for whom a lower pole resection was done for calculous disease in the left kidney. It will be seen that during the initial part of the operation, particularly during mobilization and manipulation of the kidney, there was a rise in creatinine, phosphate, and potassium excretion and a fall

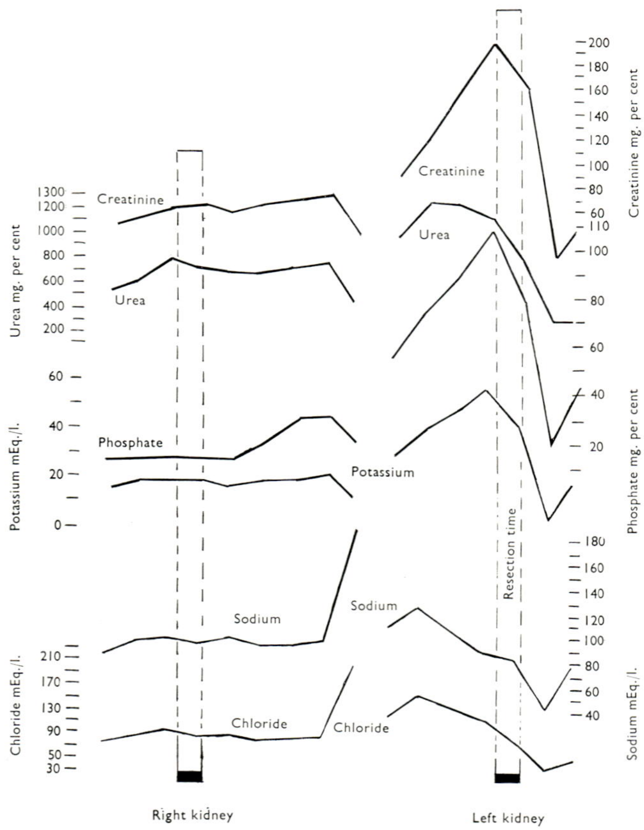

FIG. 75.—A graph of urine excretion from both kidneys during partial nephrectomy after preliminary cooling. The right kidney produced similar excretory changes to those shown in *Fig.* 74. The left kidney (subjected to operation) gave a rise in the excretion of creatinine, phosphate, and potassium in the early part of the operation when the kidney was being mobilized and manipulated, there being a fall in the sodium and chloride output. Urine excretion from the resected kidney restarted approximately 10 minutes after the clamp had been removed from the renal pedicle. There was an immediate fall of excretion of all constituents of the urine, following which there was a return to normal levels.

in sodium and chloride output. Urine excretion from the resected kidney restarted approximately 10 minutes after the clamp had been removed from the renal artery. As might be expected, there was a fall in excretion of all constituents for about 25 minutes, following which excretion rose again towards normal levels.

I believe that this technique is essential in the performance of partial nephrectomy where resection is done on the only functioning kidney. It is logical to accept that if such a technique, by reduction of biochemical disturbance and lessening of postoperative complications, can benefit a solitary kidney, then it should not be denied to the patient submitted to partial nephrectomy whose 'other kidney' is normal.

CHAPTER NINE

RESULTS OF PARTIAL NEPHRECTOMY WITH HYPOTHERMIA

By the beginning of the year 1969, partial nephrectomy under local hypothermia had been carried out on 52 patients. The age-group was wide. The youngest patient was a child of 2 years, and the oldest, a woman of 80. Of the children three were under the age of 4. As to the incidence of disease for which the operation was performed, this was approximately 40 per cent for stone, 34 per cent for hydronephrosis, 12 per cent for tuberculosis, 10 per cent for cysts and chronic abscess, and the remaining 4 per cent for hypertension and benign tumour of the kidney.

As this publication is primarily concerned with the study of the vascular pattern of the kidney and the application of this knowledge to renal surgery, there is, I think, little to be said in favour of presenting a descriptive list of all the patients who were subjected to operation. Of rather more value perhaps, is a brief note of cases of particular interest because of the complexity of their individual problem whether it was anatomical, pathological, or clinical. Of the anatomical problems, most of these presented in children or young adults, in the form of hydronephrosis. Many of these had lower segment arteries arising directly from the aorta, and passing close to the pelvi-ureteric junction, which at first sight appeared to constrict the urinary outflow. Although the results of division of the vessel and resection of the lower pole of the kidney have been good, I am not convinced that the 'aberrant' vessel is the cause of the trouble—this, however, is another story. One of the children, in whom hypothermia was essential, was a girl of 12 years old, who had hydronephrosis in a solitary kidney, the other kidney being congenitally absent. Another child, a boy of 7 years, presented with a staghorn calculus in one kidney and an associated chronic urinary infection. He also had an imperforate anus for which a colostomy had been done at birth. The other kidney was normal as shown on an intravenous pyelogram. A partial nephrectomy was done removing the staghorn calculus; the urinary infection cleared up. Some years later he returned with further urinary trouble, and on re-investigation it was found that the left kidney, which had previously been quite normal, had now become functionless, due to a recently developed urinary reflux, not from the bladder, but from a neuromuscular block at the junction of the middle and lower thirds of the left ureter. The child was therefore living entirely on the morsel of the original right kidney which had been left after partial nephrectomy for removal of the staghorn calculus.

A woman of 21 presented with a staghorn calculus in her right kidney, for which a partial nephrectomy was done under local hypothermia. Two years later she brought her 2 year-old son to see me. He, too, had a staghorn calculus, but in his left kidney. He also had a partial nephrectomy under local hypothermia for removal of the staghorn calculus.

A woman of 56, who was a diabetic and weighed 18 stone, had a staghorn calculus in her only functioning kidney. The other kidney was atrophic. A partial nephrectomy under local hypothermia was done and the stone removed. The operation was done in 1961. I saw her son some weeks ago. He told me that his mother was very well and had gone to Scotland for a holiday.

It is perhaps in a case such as the following one that hypothermia is absolutely essential. A man of 48 was admitted as an emergency with bilateral staghorn calculus of considerable size, and a blood-urea of over 250 mg. per 100 ml. He also had an abscess around one kidney. At operation, the abscess and kidney contained over 1 pint of pus. The staghorn was removed by an upper pole resection, and my osteotomy technique. By the end of 5 weeks his blood-urea had fallen to 54 mg. per 100 ml. and I was then able to remove the staghorn calculus from the opposite kidney, under hypothermia and again by the osteotomy technique.

All the previous cases have illustrated the value of hypothermia when dealing with a kidney which is diseased or solitary, that is, in a state where it is imperative to disturb the biochemical activities as little as possible, in order to avoid the possibility of further renal damage, or 'renal shutdown', in a patient who has little if any renal tissue in reserve.

The next case illustrates the value of the hypothermia technique in which the renal tissue and renal reserve was perfectly adequate, but more time was needed to perform the operation on the kidney. A man of 42 was found, on pyelography, to have an early tumour in the upper pole of the kidney. At operation, I found that the tumour was small, mobile, and I thought that it could be benign, rare though benign tumours are in a man of 40 years. This presented a fair dilemma. To carry out a local resection of the upper pole and then afterwards find that the growth was malignant, was unthinkable. On the other hand to carry out a total nephrectomy, only to find afterwards that the growth was benign, was almost as bad. Hypothermia provided an answer. I carried out a partial nephrectomy under local hypothermia, with an occlusion clamp across the renal pedicle, thereby preventing tumour dissemination by the blood-stream, if the growth should prove to be malignant. In the meanwhile, and in those extra few minutes provided by the hypothermia, it was possible to confirm by frozen-section that the growth was in fact benign. The patient was able to return to the ward having lost only one-third of a kidney. If the histological section had proved to be malignant, I was prepared to remove the remaining kidney tissue with the occlusion clamp intact.

SUMMARY OF RESULTS

In the 52 cases, there were no deaths and no postoperative urological complications. Two patients, however, did have some postoperative trouble: one, who was hypertensive, had a haemorrhage on the third postoperative day, from a superficial blood-vessel in the muscle of the abdominal wall, which needed a simple ligation to control the bleeding. The other patient developed a postoperative collapse of the lung on the same side as the operation.

FINAL COMMENT

In writing these last few paragraphs one is in a position, rather like that of 'the man who stood at the Gate of the Year', of looking back to mark the highlights of the work that was done. Of the scientific facts, there was the discovery that in the human there is a constant segmental arrangement and distribution of the arteries within the solid substance of the kidney. On the basis of this arterial distribution, the renal parenchyma is divided into five segments, which have been named the apical, upper, middle, lower, and posterior—each of which is supplied by its own artery. Although the presence of the arterial segments, within the substance of the kidney, does not change (apart from some degree in size), there is some variation in the course and exact point of origin from the renal artery or aorta of these segmental vessels outside the substance of the kidney.

When viewed on a broader scale it has been shown that there is a gradual change of pattern of these variations in the normal kidney, to the variations of the segmental arteries in the congenitally abnormal kidney—thus establishing the close relationship in the manner of their blood-supply. Likewise, study of the embryology of the mesonephric arteries provides an explanation for these variations. The nature of the segmental arteries, even in the extremes of the congenital abnormality, is the same as in the normal kidney—that is, there is no collateral circulation between these segments.

In contrast to the arteries, the venous system of the kidney presents no segmental distribution of any kind, for there is a free anastomosis from one end of the kidney to the other, by a series of intercommunicating venous arcades.

In carrying the study of these blood-vessels further in order to see the effects of disease upon them, the most noteworthy fact is the difference in the appearance of the cortical vessels, produced by a malignant tumour as distinct from a benign cyst—for in the case of the tumour, the cortical vessels, both small and large, are destroyed in the neighbourhood of the growth, whereas in the benign cyst, the segmental vessels are merely displaced and the fine vessels of the glomeruli are evident right up to the edge of the cyst.

In the study of calculous disease further support is provided for the contention that many renal calculi commence their early life as small concretions in the cortex of the kidney (possibly in the lymphatics or the tubules) which eventually migrate 'across country' of the renal cortex, to erupt into one or other of the collecting calices, from whence they may either pass out or stay and grow as does the stalagmite, by further deposition of urinary salts.

As the study of the vessels proceeded it became evident that if resection of renal tissue was to be done with the same meticulous technique employed in the resection of pulmonary tissue, then a considerable amount of time would be necessary for the operation, in order to guard against the postoperative complications of haemorrhage and urinary leakage from the cut surface of the kidney. This problem led to the idea that if the cells of the renal cortex could be induced into a temporary state of hibernation by cooling, then the anoxia would be reduced and more time would become available to carry out the operation in a bloodless field produced by occlusion of the renal artery.

Study was therefore made of the physiological effects produced by occlusion of the renal artery, whilst the kidney was subjected to cooling, down to a temperature of 17° C. Biochemical studies were made of both blood and urine, particularly of the levels and excretion of potassium, sodium, creatinine, phosphates, urea, and chlorides.

Of the clinical work, perhaps the most valuable contribution has been the application of the anatomical and physiological knowledge to operative surgery particularly in partial or segmental resection of the kidney, and by a further development of this technique for the removal of staghorn calculi.

Lastly, as there were no deaths and no urological complications following 52 operations in which partial nephrectomy was performed under local hypothermia, it is reasonable to assume that the use of hypothermia has been a valuable aid in reducing postoperative complications in this operation. I believe that the use of hypothermia *is essential* in the performance of partial nephrectomy when resection is done *on the only functioning kidney*. It is, I think, also logical to accept that if such a technique, by reduction of biochemical disturbance and the lessening of postoperative complications, can benefit a solitary kidney, then it should not be denied to the patient submitted to partial nephrectomy, whose 'other kidney' is normal.

The 'last word' is this: I believe that a nephrectomy, a total removal of one kidney, should *never* be done if a lesser procedure can offer a prospect. No one can look into the future, least of all the surgeon, and my experience has been that it is upon some tiny fragment of functioning renal tissue, left behind by partial nephrectomy, that the patient's life may ultimately depend.

Behind many stories there is a moral. If there is one here, it is, I think, that every fragment of healthy, functioning renal tissue, be it actual or potential, should be preserved providing that it has an arterial supply, a venous drainage, and a urinary exit, and that the study of anatomy has shown how this fragment may be preserved.

THE EPILOGUE

Yet to good wine they do use good bushes;
And good plays prove the better by the help of good epilogues.
As You Like It

It would not have been possible for me to have carried out this work of research, without the help of others. Wherever I have been, be it here at Stafford, in the surrounding hospitals of the Midlands, or in the teaching hospitals of University College Hospital and King's College Hospital, London, I have always received kindly co-operation, interest, and not infrequently considerable enthusiasm, from those with whom I have worked.

Unfortunately, it is not possible to mention by name everyone to whom my thanks are due, and I hope that those who receive no specific mention will not be offended, but will realize that I am nonetheless grateful to them, and that their help and kindness has not been forgotten.

There are those to whom I owe a special word of gratitude:—

To Sir Eric Riches, who has not only been kind enough to write the Prologue of this book, but who has been to me a guide and friend, in the fullest senses of the words, for he has championed my work from its earliest days, when I was a Registrar. I am particularly grateful for this, for although I have never worked for him personally, he has always accorded to me that kindly personal interest as if I had been one of his own team.

To Sir Cecil Wakeley, Bart., I would also express my thanks, for in the years that I was his Senior Registrar at King's, he gave me constant encouragement and interest, and also much kindly help in overcoming various problems.

To Professor R. S. Pilcher, I am grateful, for, in 1953, when Registrar posts in Teaching Hospitals were few and difficult to obtain, he gave me a corner of a laboratory bench on which to work and, perhaps what was more important still, a salary, for 'the bread of life', for a few additional months in order that I might complete the first phase of the work which I had set out to do.

I wish to acknowledge the help of Dr. Frank Pick of Stafford, Dr. A. J. McCall, F.R.C.P., of Stoke-on-Trent, Professor Francis Camps of the London Hospital, and Dr. B. S. Cardell and Dr. R. G. Rushton of King's College Hospital, London, and also that of many other pathologists in London and the Midlands, who so kindly gave me access to post-mortem material.

I acknowledge the kind permission of the Editor of the *British Journal of Surgery*, and also the Editor of the *Journal of Anatomy*, to reproduce illustrations and material from articles of mine which have appeared in those journals.

My thanks must also go to Mr. John Bridger, F.R.C.S., who has acted as 'critic and proof-reader'; also, to Miss Eileen Chatfield and my secretary, Mrs. Susan Bailey, who have produced the typed scripts; likewise, to the Laboratory and Theatre Staff of the Staffordshire General Infirmary who have always responded to my requests for aid, with promptness, understanding, and no doubt, at times, forbearance.

For the photographs that illustrate this book I have received help and advice from a number of people, but particularly from four sources. First, the Mid-Staffordshire Hospital Management Committee have kindly borne the financial cost of the production of special prints necessary for the manufacture of the colour-printing blocks. Secondly, Mr. Bertram Sinkinson, O.B.E., Hon. F.R.P.S., and a former President of the Royal Photographic Society, who has given much of his skill in the production of these prints. Thirdly, from Dr. J. MacDonald Holmes, F.R.C.P., who photographed the various stages of the application of hypothermia to partial nephrectomy in the operation theatre.

Lastly, but by no means least, I wish to thank my son John, in the sixth form of Downside School, for the numerous days in the school holidays of last year that he spent in the darkroom, or in the making of many of the photographs which illustrate this book. He gave of his time unstintingly, and was content with nothing less than perfection.

Finally, I wish to thank my wife. Although she has played no part in the research itself, in the early days she bore without demur the frequent hours that I spent in the laboratory, both at week-ends and at night. In the latter years, she has shown that subtle blend of cajolery, persuasion, and, at times, downright direction that all good wives use, to keep their menfolk up to standard. Indeed, without her aid, I doubt if this work would ever have been done, or this book have gone to press.

FREDERICK GRAVES

Stafford
January, 1970

REFERENCES

ABESHOUSE, B. S., and LERMAN, S. (1950), *Surgery Gynec. Obstet.*, **91,** 209.
ALBARRAN, J. (1909), *Médecine operatoire des Voies urinaires*, p. 42. Paris: Masson.
ANSON, B. J., CAULDWELL, E. W., PICK, J. W., and BEATON, L. E. (1948), *J. Urol.*, **60,** 732.
BIRKELAND, S., VOGT, A., KROG, J., and SEMB, C. (1956), *Int. physiol. Congr.*, p. 98.
BRODEL, M. (1901), *Bull. Johns Hopkins Hosp.*, **12,** 13.
BROWN, R. K. LEE (1924), *Archs Surg., Chicago*, **8,** 842.
CARR, R. J. (1954), *Br. J. Urol.*, **26,** 105.
EBERHART, C. A., and BANKS, R. (1952), *Am. Surg.*, **18,** 684.
EDSMAN, G. (1954), *Acta radiol.*, **42,** 26.
EUSTACHIUS, B. (1552), *See* LANCISI, G. M.
FELIX, W. (1912), *Human Embryology* (ed. KEIBEL and MALL), vol. 2, *Fig.* 572 and p. 822. Philadelphia: Lippincott.
GERARD, G. (1911), *J. Anat. Physiol., Paris.* **47,** 531.
GRAVES, F. T. (1954), *Br. J. Surg.*, **42,** 132.
— — (1956a), *Ibid.*, **43,** 605.
— — (1956b), *J. Anat.*, **90,** 553.
— — (1957), *Proc. R. Soc. Med.*, **50,** 368.
— — (1960), *Med. Press*, **244,** 500.
— — (1963), *Br. J. Surg.*, **50,** 362.
— — (1969), *Ibid.*, **56,** 533.
HELLSTRÖM, J. (1927), *Acta chir. scand.*, **61,** 289.
HUNTER, J. (1794), *Inflammation and Gun Shot Wounds*, p. 184. London: G. Nicol.
LANCISI, G. M. (ed.) (1714), In *Tabulae Anatomicae.* Rome.
RANDALL, A. (1937), *Ann. Surg.*, **105,** 1022.
REAGAN, G. W., and CARROLL, G. (1951), *J. Urol.*, **66,** 467.
RICHES, E. W. (1960), *Recent Advances in Surgery* (ed. SELWYN TAYLOR), ch. 12. London: Churchill.
SCHÜCK, O., HRADIC, E., FABICEN, F., and SVOBODOVA, E. (1960), *Br. J. Urol.*, **32,** 204.
SELDINGER, S. I. (1953), *Acta. radiol.*, **39,** 368.
SEMB, C. (1949), *Acta chir. scand.*, **98,** 457.
— — (1955), *Urol. int.*, **1,** 359.
— — (1956), *Ann. R. Coll. Surg.*, **19,** 137.
STEWART, H. HAMILTON (1952), *Ibid.*, **11,** 37.
— — (1960), *Br. J. Urol.*, **32,** 392.
TWINEM, F. P. (1940), *J. Urol.*, **44,** 599.
VAN SLYKE, D. D., PHILLIPS, R. A., HAMILTON, P. B., ARCHIBALD, R. M., DOLE, V. P., and EMERSON, K. (1944), *Trans. Ass. Am. Physns*, **58,** 119.
WALSH, A. (1951), *Br. J. Urol.*, **23,** 377.
WEINSTEIN, B. B., COUNTISS, E. H., and DERBES, V. J. (1940). *Urol. cutan. Rev.*, **44,** 137.
WHITESIDE, C. G. (1953), *Modern Trends in Urology* (ed. RICHES, E.), p. 33. London: Butterworths.

INDEX